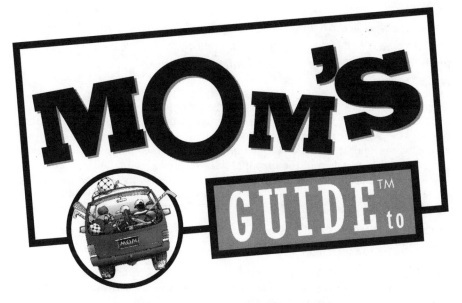

MOM'S GUIDE™ to

Your Kid's Nutrition

VICKI PORETTA
& MARCELA KOGAN

alpha books

A Division of Macmillan General Reference
A Simon & Schuster Macmillan Company
1633 Broadway, New York, NY 10019-6785

This book is dedicated to my husband, Mitchell, whose love has inspired me to become a better person, and to my young sons, Ariel and Daniel, who remind me every day why life is wonderful and precious.
—Marcela Kogan

International Standard Book Number: 0-02-861968-4

Library of Congress Catalog Card Number: 97-073176

99 98 97   4 3 2 1

Interpretation of the printing code: The rightmost number of the first series of numbers is the year of the book's printing; the rightmost number of the second series of numbers is the number of the book's printing. For example, a printing code of 97-1 shows that the first printing occurred in 1997.

Printed in the United States of America

Alpha Development Team

Brand Manager: Kathy Nebenhaus
Executive Editor: Gary M. Krebs
Managing Editor: Bob Shuman
Senior Editor: Nancy Mikhail
Development Editor: Jennifer Perillo
Editorial Assistant: Maureen Horn

Production Team

Director of Editorial Services: Brian Phair
Production Editor: Phil Kitchel
Copy Editor: Heather Stith
Illustrator: George McKeon
Designer: George McKeon
Indexer: Chris Barrick
Production Team: Cindy Fields, Linda Knose,
              Kristy Nash, Daniela Radersdorf

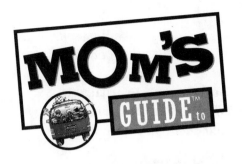

Look for these additional titles in the Mom's Guides™ series...

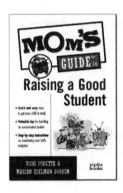

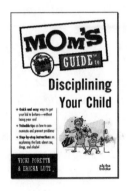

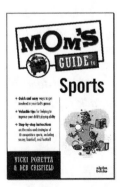

Contents

Introduction

A friend of mine told her husband that I was co-writing the *Mom's Guide to Your Kid's Nutrition*, published by the makers of the *Complete Idiot's Guide* series. "Who's going to buy that?" he asked. "Who is going to admit that they are an idiot when it comes to feeding their kids?" I said to her, "What's wrong with admitting you don't know much about nutrition?"

Are we moms supposed to understand good nutrition intuitively? Because if we are, then most of us better pack up, head back into the womb, and find crib sheets. The fact is that we have so much on our minds—work, kids, schedules, car pools, house chores, husbands—that knowing what our kids should eat is not often on the front burner.

Yet, making sure your kids eat healthful meals should be a priority, because what your kids eat today will impact their future health. Your children may seem just fine as they chow on cheeseburgers and wash the grease down with milkshakes. But what you don't see—and what should make you panic the most—is how their coronary arteries may already be starting to suffer from early stages of heart disease.

Learning to feed your kids nutritious meals just when your mind can't handle another detail may seem like an impossible task. But once you learn to select healthful foods, and get into the swing of making quick, tasty meals without a drop of sweat, you'll see that healthy meals *can* be packed into your schedule.

In this book, you will find a comprehensive guide to feeding your kids nutritious meals. You'll learn the basics of nutrition, how to read labels, and select the right foods. You'll get ideas on how to encourage finicky kids to eat, what to order when you go to restaurants, and what to feed children who have eating disorders or food sensitivities.

And, most importantly, you won't get bogged down with jargon. This book is written in plain English, so it's reader-friendly and accessible.

Making sure our kids eat healthful foods is challenging, especially as they get older and we can't keep close tabs on them. But food is an expression of love, and why not love them with all the best that nature has to offer? They'll be healthier, and you'll feel like a more accomplished parent. It's worth it—and your children's lives depend on it.

EXTRAS

Scattered throughout the text of *Mom's Guide to Your Child's Nutrition,* you'll find helpful sidebars with useful information, including helpful tips on how to make the most of meals, and danger signs that may signal health risks. Look for these features:

WISE WORDS

 This sidebar will give you definitions for foods, nutrients, and medical conditions. You don't need to become a jargon junkie to understand the world of nutrition, but learning the basic lingo will help you better grasp the fundamentals of healthful eating.

MOM KNOWS BEST

This sidebar will provide tips and shortcuts to help you understand nutritional issues, and get food on the table more quickly. You'll learn time-savings strategies so you can work, feed the family and enjoy life at the same time!

MOM ALWAYS SAID

Here, you'll find cautions and warnings you should think about when you feed your children. These sidebars will help you consider the pros and cons of buying certain foods, the importance of ensuring your kids get enough nutrients, and other suggestions.

ALL IN THE FAMILY

This sidebar supplies 'bet you didn't know' tidbits on all aspects of feeding your children nutritious meals. Anecdotes, food for thought, history and other points of interest are included.

Acknowledgments

Vicki Poretta wishes to acknowledge her husband, Joe, and their two children for their inspiration in the creation of the Mom's Guide series. Vicki also wishes to acknowledge John Rourke, Joe Fallon, and Henry Poydar of Big World Media, Inc., for their creative development and marketing of related Mom's Guide publications and products. She would also like to thank her friends at Poretta and Orr, Inc., especially Peter Laughton, for their creative help. Vicki also wishes to thank her many "sports mom" friends who lent their support and ideas along the cheering sidelines of their kids' games.

Marcela Kogan would like to thank the many editors at Macmillan Publishing for helping her develop the book. She would especially like to thank Jennifer Perillo, development editor, for her guidance, encouragement, and good spirits as the book rolled along. She was always there in all electronic formats—e-mail, fax, telephone—to support Marcela as dozens of blank pages awaited her words.

Marcela would also like to thank the women from the mom's writers group, who shared stories about feeding their children, creative ways to get finicky kids to eat, quick ways to fix healthful meals, and other tips that grounded the book in the real lives of busy moms. Thanks to Susan Glick, Meg Dennison, Louise Fisher, Renee Comet, and Pauline Steinhorn for not putting Marcela on voice-mail when she called to interview for this book.

On a special note, Marcela would also like to extend her gratitude to her brother, Sergio, 43, whose diagnosis of heart disease while she was writing the book—and subsequent triple-bypass surgery—inspired her to think longer and harder about nutrition. Many thanks also to Marcela's mother and father, for instilling a love of fruits and vegetables from the day she could chew, and to her in-laws, who took her family on vacation and watched her kids while she wrote part of her book on her laptop.

Most of all, Marcela thanks her terrific husband, Mitchell, for taking control of the household—and playing lots of UNO with their son—during the writing of the book, and for loving Marcella when she's grumpy, angry, and tired. She would also like to thank her son, Ariel, 6, who told her one day at dinner, "Mom, don't forget to write about pizza in your book," and to her lovely nine-month-old, Daniel, for sleeping through most nights so she could finish the chapters.

SPECIAL THANKS TO THE TECHNICAL REVIEWER

The *Mom's Guide to Your Kid's Nutrition* was reviewed by a dietitian who not only checked the technical accuracy of what you'll learn in this book, but also provided valuable insight to help ensure that this book tells you everything you need to know about nutrition.

Our special thanks are extended to Susan G. McDonough. Susan is currently the Diabetes Program Manager for Kaiser Permanente of the Mid-Atlantic States, Inc. Prior to that she was Manager of the Nutrition Department at Humana Group Health Plan in the Washington, D.C. metropolitan area. She is a registered, licensed dietitian. For the past 12 years she has worked as a nutritionist, counseling families on improving their nutrition to prevent, alleviate, or control various medical conditions.

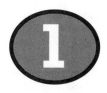

Healthy Food for the Frantic

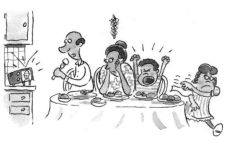

It's your turn to do carpool. You rush out of the office at 3:30, ducking your boss who has been waiting for your proposal and realizing that, once again, you forgot to thaw the chicken breasts. Another dinner of chicken nuggets—you can almost see those fried little rounds sliding down your child's throat, their fat nestling on his coronary arteries. Traffic is unusually heavy and you worry about being late. Suddenly, you noticed the red light on the gas gauge went off—your husband forgot to put gas in the car! So now, you are paranoid that your boss will fire you, your kids will get heart disease, and you'll run out of gas with a carload of kids screaming that they are hungry and need to go to the bathroom.

Will this hectic pace ever slow down? Don't count on it—at least not while your kids are still at home. We moms know nutrition is important, and many of us feel guilty that we can't make the time to cook meals over a hot stove like our own mothers did. We wonder if we are bad moms, heading down the Mommie Dearest

1

path. The answer is NO. The fact is that many of us don't know enough about nutrition: what to buy, what to serve, what our kids need.

Your child's future eating patterns depend on what he eats now, so it's worth taking the time to learn the basics of nutrition. Forget cooking over a hot stove—that's old hat. You can make quick, well-balanced meals in the microwave at a moment's notice, whip up a dinner with leftovers at the blink of an eyelash, or just bring home healthy carry-out food.

This chapter looks at how the traditional American family has changed since moms started wearing suits, highlights food guidelines everyone in the family should follow, and explains why your child's nutrition is so important.

MOMS AT WORK

While we're rushing to work, to drive our daughter to ballet class, or to get our kids' medical records for school, many of us fall into this reverie: We envision staying home, drinking juleps on our porch, and watching our kids frolic in the yard. Wake up, Mom, you've got to bring home the bacon too! And you're not alone.

Consider these statistics:

◆ Women now make up nearly half of the workforce.

◆ About 70 percent of women with children under 18 are working, up from about 45 percent two decades ago.

Many moms are trying altered work schedules so they can spend more time with the kids. Some moms work part-time or arrange flexible work schedules so they can take their kids to and from school. Others work at home, hooked up to work via fax, e-mail, and other technology.

But no matter how you look at it, the bottom line is this: Moms have less time to think about nutrition. As a result, many Americans' dinner tables look like examples of what *not* to eat to avoid heart disease. Kids dipping fried fish sticks in ketchup, pouring gobs of salt on their pasta, microwaving pizza with extra cheese and pepperoni. You know that something is wrong with this scenario, but you feel so burned out that you can't get yourself to focus. Meanwhile, your children are biting off more time from their lives every time they swallow hot dogs, cheeseburgers, and French fries.

You feel guilty? Don't bother. Guilt is out; education is in. The more you learn, the more control you'll have over your family's eating, the more confident you'll be as a parent. That's a great feeling, So sharpen your pencil, get some paper, and read on.

FOOD 101

What is food? If that question stumped you, don't get down on yourself. Eating food is one thing, but defining it is another. Basically, food is the plant and animal products our bodies must absorb in order to keep in good running condition. Foods contain, in part, the following nutrients:

♦ Carbohydrates, fats, and proteins—otherwise known as the *macro-nutrients*.

♦ Vitamins and minerals—*micro-nutrients*—ensure the right substances go to the brain, nerves, muscles, skin and bones. Minerals like calcium, for instance, are needed to form healthy bones and teeth.

If you're having flashbacks of boring high school nutrition classes, flush them out. This material isn't difficult, and we all need to know the basics to ensure that our kids grow into healthy adults. In Chapter 2, I'll explain what nutrients are and how they work in our body—so hang in there. In the meantime, it's enough to know that children need the right amount of all these nutrients. Too much or too little of any of them can cause your kid to get sick.

To give your child the right balance of nutrients, you need to know what's in the foods you serve. You can't always tell by just looking at the food. Muffins, for instance, may seem healthy because they aren't brownies. But although a bran muffin may have more nutrients than a cookie, it also tends to have lots of fat.

You can tell whether a food is healthy or not by examining the food label and purchasing products that are low-fat, low-sodium, rich in carbohydrates and have high percentages of vitamins and minerals. You'll learn how to read labels and skip over foods that are unhealthy in Chapter 3.

ARE AMERICANS NUTRITIONAL IDIOTS?

If you've been living on this planet for the past two decades, you've probably picked up on the fact that smoking cigarettes and drinking too much alcohol are bad for your health. But do you know what constitutes a good diet?

If you're like most people, you probably glance over the latest nutrition findings before flipping through the paper to find more interesting stories about corrupt politicians and celebrity scandals. Who can blame you? Nutrition, after all, isn't the sexiest issue in town.

To be fair, keeping tabs on what's what in the food world is difficult; it's even harder to figure out who is telling the truth about foods. For every study that proves one thing, another study disproves it. Myths abound: Chocolate and fried foods cause acne; sugar causes hyperactivity; the more protein you eat, the bigger your muscles will be. Then there are endless media debates over controversial nutrients. Do vitamins give you energy? Does aspartame (for example, Equal and NutraSweet) cause cancer? Is the popcorn at the movies really bad for us? Will someone please tell us the truth and nothing but the truth?

FEDS TO THE RESCUE

You can say a lot of bad things about the U.S. government, but it came through for us in the nutrition department. Some of the tools the USDA—the agency that regulates our food supply—has developed help us figure out what kinds of food and how much food our kids should eat—questions most of us couldn't answer to save our lives.

These food guidelines will help you make smart nutrition choices for your family:

◆ The *Recommended Dietary Allowances (RDAs)*—developed by the Institute of Medicine/National Academy of Sciences— represent the amounts of nutrients that you and your family should meet in order to stay healthy. (See Chapter 3 for more information about RDAs.)

◆ The *Dietary Guidelines* (available in the following list) describe food choices that will help you meet these recommendations.

◆ The *Food Guide Pyramid* and *Nutrition Facts* label are the educational tools that help you put the Dietary Guidelines into practice. The Pyramid translates the RDAs and Dietary Guidelines into the kinds and amounts of food to eat each day (see Chapters 2 and 3 for more information).

The key to a healthy diet is moderation, variety, and balance—not deprivation. But because most Americans don't know how to do anything moderately unless someone writes a rule about it, the USDA and the Department of Health and Human Services came up with seven guidelines for good eating:

MOM KNOWS BEST

No one diet fits all people. People need different amounts and kinds of food depending on their age, sex, body size, level of physical activity, and other conditions.

◆ Eat a variety of foods. Nutritionists have come up with about 40 different nutrients we all need to maintain our health. The best way to get the right amounts of each is to eat a variety of foods from each of the five basic food groups, outlined in the Pyramid (see Chapter 2). Let your kid browse the supermarket to pick out his favorites.

◆ Maintain a healthy weight—a goal that could be reached by balancing the food your child eats with physical activity. Remember, excess weight is often associated with psychological problems. How do you tell if your daughter's weight is alright? Ask your child's pediatrician, who will probably look at the height/weight tables.

◆ Lower your intake of foods high in saturated fats and cholesterol and maintain a low-fat diet. Genetics and a diet high in calories, saturated fats, and high-cholesterol foods raise your blood cholesterol level, and high blood cholesterol levels increase your risk of heart attacks.

◆ Choose a diet with plenty of veggies, fruits, and grains. About 55 to 60 percent of the total calories your kids devour should come from healthy foods like breads, cereals, pasta, rice, potatoes, dried beans, and legumes.

◆ Use sugar in moderation. Most foods contain some type of sugar. In fact, sugar (glucose) is the body's major form of fuel and the brain's best chow. But let your kids snack frequently on high-sugar cake, cookies, candy, or dried fruits, and they'll get to know the dentist really well. Sugary foods are often high in calories as well, so your children may gain weight in addition to getting cavities. Contrary to popular belief, sugar doesn't cause diabetes, heart disease, or any other major illnesses.

◆ Use salt and sodium in moderation. Ever feel like you are crossing the Dead Sea every time you eat dinner? That's probably because many foods contain sodium, often consumed as table salt. Sodium is also a preservative and is a major ingredient in MSG (used frequently in Chinese cooking), baking soda, baking powder, and other cooking ingredients. We need a small amount of sodium to maintain our health, but too much of it promotes high blood pressure.

◆ If you drink alcoholic beverages, do so in moderation. (This guideline is geared toward adults.)

These dietary principles make sense and seem realistic. You, and your children, should try to follow them throughout your lives. Many Americans are already reducing the intake of saturated fat and sodium and increasing their consumption of complex carbohydrates, but millions more are doing nothing. Even though the guidelines encourage people to maintain a healthy body weight, obesity is still the most common nutrition problem in the U.S.

HEART DISEASE STARTS NOW

You know about the inevitable skinned knees, broken ankles, bumps, and bruises your kids are bound to get. But did you ever think that your children might be subjected to heart disease, the number one killer in the nation, because of what they are eating today? You may be thinking: Isn't heart disease something that develops much later in life after all those business power lunches, steak dinners, and birthday cakes?

The unfortunate fact is that the development of heart disease starts during childhood (as early as three years old), when our kids are introduced to the great traditional American diet: too much fat, and not enough grains, fruits, and vegetables. Who would think that while your daughter is primping for the prom and your son is kicking the soccer ball, their arteries may already have spots of fatty deposits, signaling the beginning of heart disease?

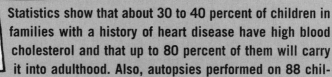

ALL IN THE FAMILY

Statistics show that about 30 to 40 percent of children in families with a history of heart disease have high blood cholesterol and that up to 80 percent of them will carry it into adulthood. Also, autopsies performed on 88 children who had died from other causes showed that almost 40 percent of them had the first signs of heart disease, which is fibrous plaque or fatty deposits in the walls of their blood vessels.

Lifetime eating habits are usually established by age eight—so now is the best time to help your kid start eating right. Remember that eating right is one step toward leading a healthy life; your child must also get exercise to keep the body in top shape. For more information about how arteries become clogged and children at risk, see Chapter 10, "Childhood Obesity."

CANCER AND DIET

Studies also point out that eating a high-fat diet can increase the risk of developing cancer, particularly colon and breast cancer. High-fat diets tend to be low in complex carbohydrates, fiber, and fruits and vegetables, which are all nutrients thought to help prevent cancer. High-fat diets are also associated with higher caloric intakes and obesity, factors that are thought to encourage the development of some cancers.

The evidence connecting some cancers to diet is so strong that the National Cancer Institute (NCI) poured millions of dollars into developing the 5 a Day for Better Health program, designed to get people to eat at least five servings of vegetables and fruits a day.

A recent NCI study on how many fruits and veggies Americans have been crunching on showed that adults are getting closer to the five-a-day goal. Their consumption went from 3.9 fruits and vegetables per day in 1991 to 4.4 in 1994. Children and teens, however, are eating 3.4 fruits and veggies a day, up only slightly from 3.1 in 1991.

Food Fraud

So how can you steer your kids away from developing heart disease, cancer, or other illnesses later in life? Truth is, a healthy, balanced diet is the only way. There are no "miracle foods" that will guarantee good health. You should be suspicious of foods that promise to cure all that ails you.

Okay, you've made it through a brief—but intense—introduction into nutrition (learning about the food pyramid, nutrients). From here on I promise lighter reading. In fact, we'll take each of these main topics and break them down so we can dive in and learn more about food and nutrition—and how you can learn to serve more balanced foods quickly at home.

THE LEAST YOU NEED TO KNOW

- ◆ Food is the plant and animal products we must eat to stay alive.

- ◆ In families with a history of heart disease, 30-40 percent of the kids have high blood cholesterol. Up to 80 percent of them will carry it into adulthood.

- ◆ Many cancers are linked to a high-fat diet.

- ◆ Nutritionists recommend that we all eat a healthy, balanced diet high in fruits, vegetables, and complex carbohydrates.

2

The ABCs of Nutrition

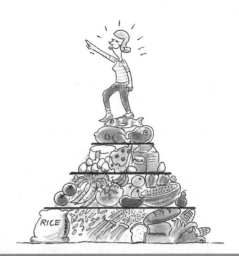

Remember when you first learned the ABCs? Let me shake the cobwebs in your brain and bring the experience back to life: Someone was teaching you the alphabet, but all you saw was a mishmash of letters that looked upside down, inside out, and flipped over. Eventually, you learned that when you put them together, you form words, and that words form sentences, and so on.

You were taking the world through your eyes—and into your hands.

Well, that's how it is with nutrition. *Proteins, carbohydrates, fiber,* and other words may sound like gobbledygook to you now. But once you learn what food is made out of and how much of what to eat to be healthy, you can take control of your nutrition—and guide your children toward leading a healthful lifestyle.

In this chapter, we're going to learn—or recap what we learned in elementary school—about the macro-nutrients, vitamins and minerals, fiber, and why we need to eat a good balance of all of them. The terminology isn't thrilling, but stick with it because learning this stuff could mean the difference between living a healthy life or heading down the road to heart disease.

THE USDA PYRAMID: BRICKS AND MORTAR FOR EATING RIGHT

The Food Guide Pyramid, the colorful Egyptian triangle created by the United States Department of Agriculture (USDA) in 1992, lays out a general guideline of what you and your family should eat to remain healthy and avoid most heart disease. You've seen it a zillion times on cereal boxes, pasta packages, and milk containers. But have you ever applied it to your child's diet?

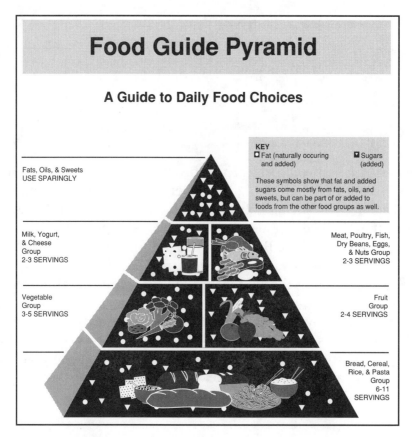

Food Guide Pyramid

A Guide to Daily Food Choices

KEY
☐ Fat (naturally occuring and added)   ■ Sugars (added)

These symbols show that fat and added sugars come mostly from fats, oils, and sweets, but can be part of or added to foods from the other food groups as well.

Fats, Oils, & Sweets
USE SPARINGLY

Milk, Yogurt, & Cheese Group
2-3 SERVINGS

Meat, Poultry, Fish, Dry Beans, Eggs, & Nuts Group
2-3 SERVINGS

Vegetable Group
3-5 SERVINGS

Fruit Group
2-4 SERVINGS

Bread, Cereal, Rice, & Pasta Group
6-11 SERVINGS

The USDA food guide pyramid.

The USDA says everyone over two years old should eat a variety of foods from five food groups every day to get the nutrients and calories they need to stay healthy:

- **Grains** (breads, cereals, rice, and pasta)**:** 6 to 11 servings

- **Vegetables:** 3 to 5 servings

- **Fruits:** 2 to 4 servings

- **Dairy products:** 2 to 3 servings

- **Meat, poultry, fish, dry beans, eggs, and nuts:** 2 to 3 servings

In addition, the USDA recommends that everyone limit their intake of fats, oils, and sweets.

Yeah, right, you're thinking, I can probably get my kids to meet the grain group requirements with pizza and pasta. But get them to eat five vegetables and four servings of fruit (which does not include fruit roll-ups)? No way!

Before you hurl this book into the trash and head out to McDonald's, hear me out. The Pyramid people know what they're talking about. The professionals who slaved over this terrific triangle made your life easier by figuring out what foods your child needs and how much of each she should eat daily. This way, you don't have to take a leave of absence from your job to figure it out yourself.

Counting Calories

Because the Pyramid's serving size ranges are so broad, you need to figure out how many servings of each food group your child needs. This amount will be based on her caloric requirements, which depend on her age, sex, size, and exercise level. Ask your doctor what your child's caloric intake should be, or follow the National Academy of Science recommendations:

- Sedentary women and some older adults need 1,600 calories a day.

- Children, teenage girls, active women, and sedentary men need 2,200 calories a day.

- Teenage boys, active men, and very active women need 2,800 calories a day.

Although it's helpful to keep these guidelines in mind, don't feel that you have to compute calories. Counting calories is a tedious, and generally unnecessary, task. A nutritionist told me she once had a patient, a healthy kid, whose mother wanted to tally calories. "I thought she was out of her mind," she told me. "It's obsessive behavior. For the run-of-the-mill mom, it's a cumbersome task." Number crunching is recommended only if your child is obese or if you have a family history of people dying young of heart attacks. (I'll talk about counting calories in Chapter 3, "This Label Could Save Your Life.")

But if your child is growing normally you don't need to worry about calories. Use the growth curve to see where your child falls, or just ask your doctors if your kid's weight is right for her size, age, and sex.

Remember that kids need more calories than adults because a major chunk of their growth takes place during adolescence. That's when they suddenly sprout and begin towering over you, and you find yourself saying, "Is that you? I can't believe it!"

How Many Servings Does Your Kid Need?

The Pyramid nutritionists came up with a recommended number of food group servings for each of the three calorie levels. Teenage girls and children, who need 2,200 calories a day, should eat the following number of servings:

- Nine servings from the grain group

- Four servings from the vegetable group

- Three servings from the fruit group

◆ Two to three servings from the milk group

◆ Two servings from the meat, poultry, and fish group

Teenage boys (who need 2,800 calories a day), should eat the following number of servings:

◆ Eleven servings from the grain group

◆ Five servings from the vegetable group

◆ Four servings from the fruit group

◆ Three servings from the milk group

◆ Three servings from the meat, poultry, and fish group

Serving Sizes

So, what's a serving? One guy I know considers a bag of Oreos, which he polishes off in one sitting, one serving. If everyone creates their own serving portions, the Pyramid is pretty worthless. But when the feds at the USDA created the Pyramid, they definitely had portions in mind. For example, half of a cup of pasta, a measly amount, equals one serving. A serving of meat is only two to three ounces. (You can forget the 12-ounce filet.) Every time your kid eats a slice of bread, he's getting one serving from the grain group.

According to the *USDA's Dietary Guidelines for Americans*, 1995, the following amounts count as servings.

Grain group (bread, cereal, rice, and pasta):

◆ One slice of bread

◆ One ounce of ready-to-eat cereal

◆ Half a cup of cooked cereal, rice, or pasta

Vegetable group:

◆ One cup of raw leafy vegetables

◆ Half of a cup of other vegetables, cooked or raw

◆ Three-fourths of a cup of vegetable juice

Fruit group:

◆ One medium apple, banana, or orange

◆ Half of a cup of chopped, cooked, or canned fruit

◆ Three-fourths of a cup of fruit juice

Dairy group (milk, yogurt, and cheese):

◆ One cup of milk or yogurt

◆ One and a half ounces of natural cheese

◆ Two ounces of processed cheese

Meat and beans group (meat, poultry, fish, dry beans, eggs and nuts):

◆ Two to three ounces of cooked lean meat, poultry, or fish (Half of a cup of cooked dry beans or one egg counts as one ounce of lean meat. Two tablespoons of peanut butter or one-third of a cup of nuts count as one ounce of meat.)

MOM KNOWS BEST

If your child doesn't enjoy eating foods from a particular group (like vegetables), throw ingredients together and get more bang for your buck. A slice of pizza, for instance, counts in the grain group (crust), the milk group (cheese), and the vegetable group (tomato). You can even add veggies on top for extra nutrition. You know your kid is gulping down some serious servings, but all he knows is that he doesn't have to have another cup of yogurt.

When your kid eats isn't as important as what he eats. Be flexible. If your kid eats lots of healthful snacks, serve him fewer portions during mealtimes. Or if he likes to eat mostly at meals, give him larger servings then. Don't panic if he doesn't eat the right amount of servings from each food group every day. Kids tend to eat balanced meals in fits and starts. As long as he eats something from each food group over several days, that's fine.

CHEMISTRY 101: PROTEIN, CARBOS, FAT, VITAMINS, AND MINERALS

You may never have thought of this before, but all the foods you eat contain carbohydrate, protein and fat. Some food are made up mostly of carbohydrates (like pasta). While others, like pizza, combine all three in one bite! This terrific trio is called macro-nutrients because your body needs all of them in different amounts to work well.

Your kid's diet should consist of 55 to 60 percent carbohydrates, 10 to 15 percent protein, and less than 30 percent fat—of which no more than 10 percent should be saturated fat.

Carbohydrates, protein, and fat, which are called *macronutrients*, are the big kids on the block; they provide your child with the calories she needs to live a healthy life. Vitamins and minerals are smaller players in the good health game, but they are still essential for normal body functions and growth.

With a nutritious diet, the carbohydrate, protein, and fat sources your child eats will supply her body with 13 vitamins and at least 22 minerals. Their job is to regulate her metabolism, convert fat and carbohydrates to energy, and help form her bones and tissues. The following sections explain what you need to know about these building blocks of nutrition.

PROTEINS: THE STUFF OF LIFE

Proteins are the guys your kid wants on her team when she tears a ligament, gets an infection, or feels that her digestive system is out of whack. These molecules help build new tissues and replace old ones, produce antibodies to help fight infection, and carry oxygen through the blood. Without proteins, your child is more susceptible to disease.

Each protein molecule is made up of subunits called *amino acids*. Twenty different amino acids are found in body proteins, all of which carry nitrogen, an element needed for human life. Our bodies make 11 amino acids, and the rest, called *essential amino acids*, come from the foods we eat. Your kid can't make them, but she's gotta have them. Where does she get them? She gets them from animal proteins, including meat, fish, poultry, cheese, and eggs.

These foods are called *complete proteins* because they carry all the essential amino acids we need.

WISE WORDS

Proteins are compounds made up of carbon, hydrogen, oxygen, and nitrogen which are necessary for life. Next to water, our bodies are made up primarily of proteins.

Amino acids are the building blocks of the proteins your body needs. Your diet must provide nine necessary amino acids; your body produces the rest (11 of them).

Essential amino acids are the nine necessary amino acids found in animal protein that the body can't make on its own and must rely on outside food sources to obtain.

If your child doesn't eat meat, don't despair. You can also find protein in vegetable products, such as grains, legumes, nuts, seeds, and other vegetables. The problem is that these vegetables don't have all the amino acids in tow. And if one or two amino acid guys are missing from the chain, the rest might as well go home because they can't do their job. To bring all the amino amigos together, combine the vegetables with grains.

Here's where you can get creative: If grains and legumes turn your kid on, let her gobble up complete proteins by giving her a peanut butter sandwich on whole-wheat bread, rice and beans, or vegetarian chili with bread.

If she's into the grain and nut/seed combo, give her some rice cakes with peanut butter or a whole-wheat bun with sesame seeds. Another way to ensure she gets complete proteins is to give her foods from the legumes and nuts/seed combination, such as humus (chickpeas and sesame paste) and trail mix (a mixture of peanuts and sunflower seeds).

Your child has to eat protein every day, because her body can't store it. The federal government recommends a diet consisting of 10 to 15 percent protein. To find out how many grams of protein your child needs daily, multiply her weight by .36 grams. Example: If she weighs 60 pounds, she needs about 21.6 grams of protein per day (60 × .36).

Getting enough protein is rarely a problem. Your child, for instance, can meet (and exceed) her daily protein requirement by eating one 3½- to 4-ounce steak (26 grams of protein). If she's a vegetarian, she can eat an ounce of American cheese (six grams of protein), an ounce of peanuts (12 grams of protein), and a yogurt (12 grams of protein) to meet her daily needs.

Make sure you choose healthy sources of protein for your child. Red meat, for example may be rich in protein, but it is also high in fat and cholesterol. Compare the following:

◆ A three-ounce portion of lean ground beef (20 grams of protein) has 15.7 grams of fat, 6.2 g of saturated fats, and 74 mg of cholesterol.

◆ Three ounces of chicken breast without skin (26 grams of protein) has 3 grams of fat, .9 g of saturated fats, and 58 mg of cholesterol.

◆ A three-ounce portion of flounder (19 grams of protein) has 1.3 g total fat, .3 g saturated fats and 58 mg of cholesterol

Clearly, your child should eat red meat in moderation. Before cooking, be sure to trim the fat off of meats and remove the skin from poultry. And remember: All these figures will change depending on how you cook the food and how large your portions are.

But don't grab the hot dog off your child's plate yet. The key to eating well is moderation. Over the course of a week, you could serve at least one fish meal, a couple of chicken dishes, and no more than two lean red meat platters.

The Protein Content of Common Foods	
FOOD	*PROTEIN (IN GRAMS)*
Ground beef, 3 oz., broiled	21 grams
Ham, 3 oz., roasted	18 grams
Beef tenderloin, 3 oz., broiled	22 grams
Chicken, 3.5 oz., roasted	27 grams
Turkey, 3.5 oz., roasted	28 grams

continues

The Protein Content of Common Foods *(continued)*

FOOD	PROTEIN (IN GRAMS)
Salmon, 3.5 oz., baked or broiled	27 grams
Flounder, 3.5 oz., baked	30 grams
Tuna, 3.5 oz., canned in water	28 grams
Scallops, 3.5 oz., steamed	18 grams
Beef bologna, 1 oz.	3 grams
Beef frankfurter	6 grams
Chicken roll, 1 oz.	6 grams
Milk, 1 cup (whole, low-fat, or skim)	8 grams
Yogurt, 8 oz., low-fat, plain	12 grams
Cheese, 1 oz., cheddar	7 grams
Eggs, 1 large, boiled	6 grams
Cottage cheese, 1/2 cup, low-fat	15.5 grams

Source: USDA

Proteins are found nearly everywhere in our bodies—our bones, organs, tendons, muscles, hair, and skin. And they have a lot to do: They make sure chemical reactions take place, help fight disease, carry oxygen all over the body, repair body tissue, and carry out other tasks.

But if your kid is devouring protein like crazy because he thinks extra protein will help him build larger muscles, you better break it to him. Excessive protein is needed to develop muscle but it won't build bigger biceps. For that, he has to exercise. And what happens to all the extra protein? It goes down the toilet.

CARBOHYDRATES: UH-OH, SPAGHETTI-OS!

If it weren't for cereal, what would your children eat? One mom told me that her son eats cereal three times a day: cereal and milk for breakfast, cereal for desert at lunch, and cereal as a side dish for dinner. No doubt, he's getting a good share of his daily carbohydrates.

Carbohydrates are the body's main energy source. The Recommended Daily Allowance (RDA) of carbohydrates for school-age kids is about 53 percent of the total calories consumed daily. So if your child is on a 2,200-calorie diet, she should take in about 1,200 calories in carbohydrates.

There are two kinds of carbohydrates. *Simple carbohydrates*, also called *simple sugars*, are sweet and sticky products like honey, candy, and soft drinks. Most simple sugars are empty calories because they don't provide the body with anything nutritional. Fruit and milk, are made up largely of simple sugars, but they contain many vitamins so their calories are not "empty." A Coke has calories, but no nutritional value, but a glass of orange juice gives calories plus Vitamin C. *Complex carbohydrates*, which consist of hundreds of simple sugars linked together, include pasta, breads, cereals, rice, and beans. Carbohydrates that come from plants are called *starches* and are found in grains, vegetables, and legumes.

Complex carbohydrates take quite a beating in your digestive tract, as *enzymes* (protein molecules that act as catalysts for chemical reactions) hack away at them until they turn into their simplest form, called *glucose*. Your body recognizes this simple sugar, absorbs it, and then turns it into energy.

WISE WORDS

Carbohydrates are organic molecules made up primarily of carbon, hydrogen and oxygen atoms that supply energy to the brain, central nervous system and muscle cells.

Simple carbohydrates are the most basic kind of carbohydrate, made up of *simple sugars* like honey, jellies, soft drinks.

When many simple sugars are linked together they are called *complex carbohydrates*. Complex carbohydrates that come from plants are called starch, usually found in vegetables, breads, seeds, beans.

FATS: LOVE-HATE RELATIONSHIP

Fats: Can't live with them, can't live without them. Despite all we know about the link between high-fat diets and heart disease, studies show that on average, kids consume 35 percent of their total calories from fat. Big, juicy steaks, meatloaf with gravy, and hot fudge sundaes with whipped cream on top may have been your favorite comfort foods when you were growing up, but they shouldn't be a part of your kids' regular diet.

MOM KNOWS BEST

Limit the fat in your children's diets to 30 percent of daily calories. Children who consume 1,600 calories a day should eat no more than 53 grams of fat a day. Those who consume 2,200 calories should have less than 73 grams, and those who consume 2,800 calories can go as high as 93 grams.

Don't impose a total ban on fat, however. After all, fat makes up an important part of your kids' nutrition. Without fat as padding, our organs would jiggle around inside our bodies—a scary thought considering how much kids jump around. Fat also protects us from being too cold or hot and keeps our hair and skin from being too dry.

Crazy Over Cholesterol

The problem with high-fat foods is that, in addition to having too many calories, many are loaded with *saturated fats*, which are substances that raise *blood cholesterol* and pave the way for heart disease. Saturated fat looks like the stuff on top of the gravy boat that your mother told you to never pour down the drain. Imagine this hardened grease clogging up your arteries, and you'll understand why this fat is so threatening.

Our bodies make *cholesterol*, a waxy substance which contributes to the formation of many essential compounds (including vitamin D, bile acid, estrogen, and testosterone), to perform vital functions. Our livers make all the cholesterol we need, and the unused portion all too often gets stored as *plaque* in our arteries.

Pediatricians urge parents who have a family history of heart disease to get their children's cholesterol checked. The American Academy of Pediatrics recommends that children under 19 have total cholesterol levels (including the good and bad cholesterol—see the Wise Words) below 170 mg/dl. If your child's cholesterol level is higher, cut down on fats, particularly saturated fats. If your child is eating about 2,800 calories a day, for example, try to limit the amount of fat calories to 784 (30 percent of 2,800) or 87 grams. The amount of saturated fat in his diet shouldn't exceed 84 calories, or about 9 grams.

WISE WORDS

A waxy substance that helps form essential compounds including adrenal and sex hormones, bile acids, and vitamin D in the skin, *cholesterol* is carried in the blood along in three types of *lipoproteins*: low-density, very low-density, and high-density. Your body produces all the cholesterol you need, and the excess gets stored as plaque in your arteries.

High-density lipoprotein (HDL), the "good" cholesterol, helps your body get rid of blood cholesterol.

Low-density lipoprotein (LDL), the "bad" cholesterol, builds up in the walls of your arteries. The higher your LDL cholesterol, the greater your risk for heart problems.

The devil of all fats, *saturated fats* are responsible for raising your blood cholesterol and paving the way to heart disease.

MOM KNOWS BEST

It's important to understand the difference between dietary cholesterol (what you consume in food) and blood cholesterol (what circulates in the blood). When doctors say you have high cholesterol, they mean you have too much cholesterol in your bloodstream—a problem that leads to fatty deposits in the coronary arteries. Cholesterol-rich foods can raise blood cholesterol, but foods with huge amounts of saturated fats can raise it even more.

Your kid can consume 87 grams of fat without even trying. A bologna and cheese sandwich made with two slices of meat, two slices of cheese, and two teaspoons of mayonnaise equals 36 grams of fat, and that's just one sandwich! You can help reduce your child's fat intake by making healthier alternatives. For instance, a lean beef sandwich made with lettuce, tomato, and low-fat mayonnaise served with a cup of nonfat milk has only 6 grams of fat.

Getting Off the Trans-Fatty Acids Express

Try also to avoid eating foods that contain *trans-fatty acids* (foods like tub or stick margarine). Trans-fatty acids are created through a hydrogenation process in which liquid or semi-soft fat is transformed into a more solid silly putty state. These acids can contribute to heart disease because they act like saturated fats inside the body and raise blood cholesterol. And they sound so yucky! If I were you, I wouldn't bother learning more about the hydrogenation process unless you have a tough stomach.

But if you want to be on the safe side, choose margarine listing liquid oil as the first ingredient.

WISE WORDS

Trans-fatty acids are created when unsaturated fats go through a manufacturing process called hydrogenation. A normally soft or liquid polyunsaturated fatty acid is transformed into a harder, more saturated fat—and the body treats it like it would a saturated fat. Why saturate? One reason foodmakers do it is to preserve foods.

Unsaturated Fats

Unsaturated fats, on the other hand, are much kinder to your body. They include *monounsaturated fats* (olive oil, peanut oils, and canola oil) that liquefy at room temperature and come from vegetable sources. Studies show that these fats may help lower blood cholesterol, but if you are watching your kid's weight, make sure you use monounsaturated fats sparingly since they are full of fat calories.

Polyunsaturated fats, such as corn oils, cottonseed oils, safflower oils, and soybean oils, have also been shown to help reduce the risk of heart disease. The "omega-3" oils, a type of polyunsaturated fat found in tuna, salmon, mackerel and other fatty fish, tend to act as a blood thinner, keeping plaque from forming around the arteries.

WISE WORDS

Unsaturated fats are composed of either *mono-unsaturated fats*, typically found in olive oils, peanut oils, sesame seed oils, canola oils, and avocadoes, or *poly-unsaturated fats* from corn, soybean, safflower, sunflower and sesame seed oils.

VITAMINS: GREAT FOR GROWTH

Don't underrate the jobs performed by vitamins and minerals—the micro-nutrients—just because carbohydrates, fat and protein steal the headlines. After all, vitamins and minerals work hard behind the scenes to build red blood cells, develop and maintain body tissues and do other tasks to make sure the macro-nutrients can shine and the person can grow well.

Here is how the micros and macros work together: Your child eats carbohydrates, proteins and fat, which supply his body with the 13 vitamins and at least 22 minerals. If one mineral or vitamin punches out early, another nutrient that does the same thing must replace it for your child to feel healthy.

Vitamins are divided into two groups: *Fat-soluble* (vitamins A, D, E, and K) and *water-soluble* (eight B vitamins and vitamin C).

The fat-soluble vitamins are stored in your body's fat. Without vitamin D, for instance, your child can get bone abnormalities, including rickets. Be careful, though—too many of these vitamins can be a bad thing. Too much vitamin A intake, for instance, can cause a potentially deadly condition known as "retinoid toxicity" in which bones begin to lose minerals rapidly, and hair and skin are shed. If your child takes in too much vitamin D, he or she can get too much calcium in the blood.

WISE WORDS

Vitamins A, D, E, and K are *fat-soluble*, or transported into the bloodstream by fats. Taking too many of these vitamins could be harmful.

Water-soluble vitamins are stored and carried by the water in our system. Because we lose a lot of water through urine and other body fluids, most of these vitamins must be replaced daily. Water-soluble vitamins include vitamin C and the many B-complex vitamins.

How can you tell if your kid is getting too much of a good thing?

Just keep an eye on the nutrition label, which will tell you what percentage of the daily value for major vitamins one serving of that food contains, based on a 2,000 calorie diet. Turn to Chapter 3 to learn how to read labels.

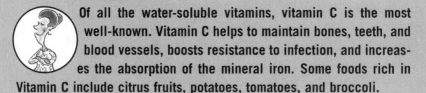

MOM KNOWS BEST

Of all the water-soluble vitamins, vitamin C is the most well-known. Vitamin C helps to maintain bones, teeth, and blood vessels, boosts resistance to infection, and increases the absorption of the mineral iron. Some foods rich in Vitamin C include citrus fruits, potatoes, tomatoes, and broccoli.

If you're worried that your child isn't getting enough vitamins, talk to your child's pediatrician before giving your child a supplement. In some cases, the pediatrician may recommend vitamin supplements. If, for example, your kid is a vegan (the strictest type of vegetarian who eats no animal products at all), vitamin B12 supplements are essential. (This type of diet, some say, is dangerous for growing children.) But vitamin deficiencies are rare in the U.S. Most kids get all the vitamins they need in their diet.

Foods rich in vitamins include the following:

◆ Milk fortified with vitamins A and D

◆ Eggs

◆ Dark green leafy vegetables

◆ Fruits

◆ Whole-grain enriched cereals and breads (for the B vitamins especially)

If your kid is eating these foods regularly, don't worry that he isn't getting enough vitamins.

In general, the way to provide children with adequate vitamins is to give them a varied diet. Avoid overcooking foods, which may destroy certain vitamins. Steaming vegetables is a good way to retain vitamins. Refrigeration and freezing also preserve vitamins in many fruits and vegetables.

MINING THE MINERALS YOU NEED

Vitamins and minerals are interchangeable, right? Wrong. Minerals are *inorganic substances* (they don't contain carbon) that are crucial to keeping hundreds of body processes going on. Minerals perform three basic functions:

◆ Calcium, phosphorus, and magnesium, for instance, are embedded in the bones, teeth, muscles, and other tissues.

◆ Many minerals are required for enzymes to function. And enzymes, in turn, are needed to get chemical reactions going in the body.

◆ Minerals called electrolytes (sodium and potassium chloride) balance the fluids in the body and regulate the acid-base content of the blood.

A well-balanced and varied diet usually gives your child adequate minerals to replace whatever minerals are lost every day. Except for iron and maybe zinc, mineral deficiencies in healthy American children are unusual.

Your child needs 22 minerals along with vitamins to keep his internal engines running properly. He needs large amounts of major minerals, like calcium and potassium, and smaller amounts of trace-minerals like iron and zinc. Calcium is the most abundant mineral in the body—99 percent of our body's calcium is stored in the bones. Iron deficiency, however, is the most widespread type of vitamins or mineral deficiency in the world.

Bone-Building Calcium

Calcium is the most abundant mineral in the body. Your child needs calcium for healthy bone development. As mom used to say, "Drink your milk so your bones will get big and strong!" The RDA for calcium is 1,200 milligrams for children and teenagers. Children 6 to 10 should consume 800 to 1,200 milligrams. Those 11 to 24 need between 1,200 to 1,500 milligrams. Plenty of foods provide these requirements. Just three ounces of sardines, for instance, have 372 milligrams of calcium.

ALL IN THE FAMILY

Serve your kids meals with high levels of calcium, iron, thiamin, and vitamins A and C. These nutrients are lacking in many adolescent diets. The need for calcium, especially, increases at this age because the weight of the skeleton grows 45 percent as kids get 20 percent taller and 50 percent heavier. Girls' growth spurt begins at 10 or 11 and lasts until they are 15. Boys begin their spurt at 12 or 13 and end it at 19 years of age.

What? Your preteen doesn't like sardines? How about a cup of low-fat yogurt? It's worth 415 milligrams of calcium—nearly half of the RDA. Check out other calcium sources:

◆ One oz. of Monterey Jack, 207 mg

◆ ½ cup of ice cream, 88 mg

◆ One cup of whole milk, 291 mg

◆ ½ cup of cooked broccoli, 68 mg

◆ ¼ cup of raisins, 22 mg

◆ 2 Tbsp peanut butter, 18 mg,

◆ 4 oz of processed tofu with calcium 145 mg

◆ 1 oz of calcium fortified cereals (Total) with ½ cup of milk, 350 mg.

◆ An 8-oz cup of calcium-fortified orange juice, 300 mg

Pumping Up with Iron

Iron, another well-known mineral, is responsible for delivering oxygen to every cell of your child's body. You can find iron in various foods. *Heme iron*, the most absorbable type, is found in animal products such as meat, liver, poultry, seafood, and eggs. *Nonheme iron* is less absorbable and is found in dried fruits, nuts, beans, and fortified grains.

> **WISE WORDS**
>
> *Iron* deficiency is widespread. Nearly 70 to 80 percent of iron is found in hemoglobin, the oxygen carrying molecules in the red blood cells. *Heme iron* is found in animal products, like lean red meats, turkey, eggs, lamb, fish and seafood, and is more easily absorbed than *Nonheme iron*, which comes from plant sources such as beans, broccoli, spinach, and dried fruit. Because nonheme iron isn't easily absorbed, vitamin C and other acids can increase absorption.

You can boost the absorption rate of iron by combining foods high in vitamin C with an iron-rich meal (for example, try serving a breakfast of iron-fortified cereal with a glass of orange juice).

Most kids can meet their iron needs from their meals. Girls beginning to menstruate may need to eat more iron-rich foods because they lose a lot of blood each cycle.

Some examples of minerals and what they do:

- Zinc is found in more than 100 enzymes essential to digestion and metabolism.

- Potassium, along with sodium, helps to regulate the body's fluid balance. It's needed for proper metabolism.

- Sodium helps maintain body fluid balance.

- Iodine is crucial to normal thyroid-gland function.

FIRE UP WITH FIBER

We don't need fiber to live well, but it sure feels good when you gotta go. Fiber, which has no nutritional value, consists of various plant food substances that cannot be digested. Why eat something you don't need? Fiber can help reduce the risk of colon cancer, lower cholesterol, and keep your child's body regular (if you know what I mean).

There are two kinds of fiber: *water-soluble* and *water-insoluble*. Water-soluble fiber can help decrease blood cholesterol and is found in oats, brown rice, barely, vegetables, and some fruits. Insoluble fiber, found in foods such as wheat bran, cereals, and legumes, moves the bowels. Insoluble fiber helps accelerate intestinal transit time and increases and softens stools. It also decreases the risk of colon cancer and diverticulosis, a disease characterized by pouches that develop in weak areas of the large intestine, causing abdominal pain, bleeding, and diarrhea.

WISE WORDS

 Fiber has no nutritional value and humans can't digest it, but its benefits include its ability to pick up water and add bulk to the stool, which makes passage through the GI track easier.

Water-soluble fiber dissolves in water. Soluble fiber can be found in oats, barley, beans, rye, vegetables, fruits and oat bran.

Water-insoluble fiber doesn't readily dissolve and is found in foods like wheat bran, fruits, vegetables, whole-wheat breads and cereals, legumes.

To calculate how many grams of fiber your child needs, add five to your kid's age and stop at 15 grams. Your eight-year old, for instance, needs 13 grams a day. Most kids don't get enough fiber. This condition results in constipation. Those who get enough in their system often don't drink enough water, which makes them more constipated. Experts say our children need to drink more water.

WATER: LET IT FLOW

We can live without food for several weeks, but without water we might as well hang it up after a few days. Water plays a vital role in digestion, absorption of nutrients, growth and repair of tissues, removal of waste products, and other body interactions. Water also regulates body temperature and carries nutrients and oxygen to all our cells.

In fact, water makes up 92 percent of our blood, 22 percent of our bones, 75 percent of our muscles, and 75 percent of our brain. Talk about feeling water-logged! Experts are concerned about kids not drinking enough water during hot weather and becoming dehydrated. (See Chapter 8, "Jock Food," for keeping athletes hydrated).

The American Dietetic Association, along with other experts, put out some do's and don'ts for keeping kids hydrated during the summer. Some tips:

◆ Encourage them to drink at least eight glasses of water a day. Kids lose two or more quarts of water daily so their bodies need lots of water.

◆ Urge your child to take water breaks every 15-20 minutes while playing outside or doing sports—and give them a cold water bottle when they go out bike riding.

◆ When going on a weekend trip, put water in the cooler. To keep a bottle of water cold most of the day, freeze one half of a bottle before you go to sleep, and fill it up to the brim with water the next morning.

THE LEAST YOU NEED TO KNOW

◆ The Food Pyramid points out that your child must eat a variety of foods from the five food groups to be healthy.

◆ Children and teenage girls need 2,200 calories a day; teenage boys need 2,800 calories a day.

◆ Your child's diet should be made up of 55 to 60 percent carbohydrates (mostly complex carbos), 10 to 15 percent protein, and less than 30 percent fat, of which no more than 10 percent should be saturated.

◆ More than 13 vitamins and 22 minerals are crucial for your child's body to function properly.

◆ Make sure your child has calcium in his diet to enhance bone building and iron.

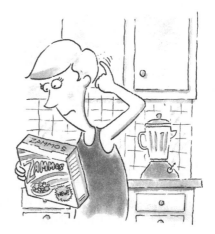

3

This Label Could Save Your Life

Congratulations, you're no longer a nutritional neophyte. Now you know which nutrients, both macro and micro, your kid needs in order to eat healthy. You no longer have to live in fear that someone will strike up a conversation about saturated fats, and you won't know what she's talking about. Your next mission, should you choose to accept it, is to learn to read food labels so that you know exactly what a product is made of and how many nutrients a serving contains.

Don't hit the supermarket aisles just yet, especially not if you've just had a long day at work. Imagine your eight-year-old sitting in the shopping cart dangerously close to the eggs and tomatoes and your preteen nagging, "Let's go!" every 15 seconds while you are trying to focus on the label. That'll drive you to the nearest fast-food window. For now, practice reading labels at home, all snuggled up in your bathrobe and slippers, by going through the products on your shelf.

WHY READ LABELS?

Looking at the Nutrition Facts label can be a frustrating, demoralizing experience—all those numbers in milligrams and grams leading to percentages. But this label can be a useful guide as you design a balanced, healthy diet.

The food label is pretty thorough. It lists every major nutrient in the food, as well as vitamins and minerals. For some consumers, it may be more than they want to know. But for others, it may not be enough. Once you know how to read a label, you'll be able to compare products, groan over fat content, gasp over sodium, and cheer for products rich in carbohydrates. How wonderful, how hip, how '90s! And once you learn how to read the nutrition label, you'll wonder how you ever got by without it.

ALL IN THE FAMILY

The Food Marketing Institute, which conducted a survey of 1,000 shoppers, found that shoppers wanted lots of information about products. Fat content was the number one interest, followed closely by ingredients, calories, and other nutrients. Although many people read the food label, others just glanced at the brand name, the expiration date, or the package weight. (Package weight? Someone has to explain that one to me.)

The label is designed for the average American who takes in about 2,000 calories a day. It is also based on a diet consisting of less than 30 percent fat (less than 65 grams), about 55 percent carbohydrates (300 grams), about 15 percent protein (15 grams), and less than 300 milligrams of cholesterol (65 grams). Keep in mind that teenagers need between 2,200 and 2,800 calories (preteens need slightly less), so adjust the nutrition information to fit your child's calorie requirements.

INSIDE NUTRITION FACTS

The nutritional information is listed not because food manufacturers want to divulge their secrets, but because the feds made them spill the beans about what's in each serving of their products. The Nutrition Labeling and Education Act of 1990 (NLEA) requires the following items:

◆ Nutritional information on almost all foods

◆ A new format for presenting nutritional information

◆ Adherence to a standard set of definitions for claims like "no fat" and "high fiber"

◆ Appropriate use of seven scientifically proven claims about the relationship between a nutrient to a medical condition

I'll get into how to read labels and decode claims later in this chapter.

Sizing Up Servings

The NLEA requires that serving sizes be more uniform and reflect the amount that people actually eat. The NLEA defines a serving size as the amount of food eaten by one person at one time.

But how true are these serving sizes? Last time I looked, a serving of pasta was half a cup. That's barely enough strands to twirl around a fork. Imagine having six people over for dinner and serving one package of pasta, which has eight two-ounce servings. For sure, someone would make a run to Taco Bell to get more food. Can you imagine your child eating one serving (half a cup) of ice cream? Let's face it—the kid will probably down two portions.

Counting Calories

The Calories item on the label refers to the amount of calories in a single serving of that food. Next to it, the Calories from Fat item tells you how many of those calories come from fat. You should limit your child's fat intake to 30 percent of her daily calories. For example, a person on a 2,000 daily caloric level should consume 600 fat calories a day (30 percent of 2,000) or 67 grams of fat.

For example, consider two products: rice cakes and chocolate chip cookies. One rice cake has 40 calories, none from fat. But three cookies have 160 calories, 70 of which come from fat. Twelve percent of all the cookie calories come from fat! The rice cakes are obviously the healthier choice, but most people would agree that the cookies are the tastier one. You might use this information to determine that rice cakes can be a part of you child's regular diet (if he'll eat them), and cookies are OK once in a while.

Nutrition Facts

Serving Size 1 Cake (10g)
Servings Per Container 14

Amount Per Serving

Calories 40

	% Daily Value*
Total Fat 0g	0%
Cholesterol 0mg	0%
Sodium 90mg	4%
Total Carbohydrate 8g	3%
Protein 1g	

Not a significant source of Calories from Fat, Saturated Fat, Dietary Fiber, Sugars, Vitamin A, Vitamin C, Calcium, Iron.

*Percent Daily Values are based on a 2,000 calorie diet.

Ingredients: Corn (with germ removed), whole grain brown rice, natural cheese flavor blend [whey, cheddar cheese* (milk, salt, cheese cultures, enzymes), salt, nonfat dry milk, buttermilk*, citric acid, natural flavors].

*Adds a negligible amount of fat.

Rice Cakes

Nutrition Facts

Serving Size 3 Cookies (32g)
Servings Per Container About 5

Amount Per Serving

Calories 160 Calories from Fat 70

	% Daily Value*
Total Fat 8g	12%
Saturated Fat 2.5g	12%
Cholesterol 0 mg	0%
Sodium 105mg	4%
Total Carbohydrate 21g	7%
Dietary Fiber 1g	3%
Sugars 10g	
Protein 2g	

Vitamin A 0%	•	Vitamin C 0%
Calcium 0%	•	Iron 4%

*Percent Daily Values are based on a 2,000 calorie diet. Your daily values may be higher or lower depending on your calorie needs:

		Calories:	2000	2500
Total Fat	Less than		65g	80g
Sat Fat	Less than		20g	25g
Cholesterol	Less than		300mg	300mg
Sodium	Less than		2400mg	2400mg
Total Carbohydrate			300g	375g
Dietary Fiber			25g	30g

Calories per gram:
Fat 9 • Carbohydrate 4 • Protein 4

INGREDIENTS: ENRICHED WHEAT FLOUR (CONTAINS NIACIN, REDUCED IRON, THIAMINE MONONITRATE [VITAMIN B₁], RIBOFLAVIN [VITAMIN B₂]), SWEET CHOCOLATE CHIPS (MADE WITH SUGAR, CHOCOLATE, COCOA BUTTER, DEXTROSE, SOY LECITHIN-AN EMULSIFIER), VEGETABLE SHORTENING (PARTIALLY HYDROGENATED SOYBEAN OIL), SUGAR, BROWN SUGAR, HIGH FRUCTOSE CORN SYRUP, LEAVENING (BAKING SODA, AMMONIUM PHOSPHATE), SALT, WHEY, NATURAL AND ARTIFICIAL FLAVOR.

Chocolate Chip Cookies

How rice cakes and chocolate chip cookies differ in calorie content, fat, saturated fat, and cholesterol.

Facing Fat

The Total Fat item on the nutrition label shows the total number of fat grams coming from saturated, monounsaturated, and polyunsaturated fats (see Chapter 2, "The ABC's of Nutrition" for definitions of the different kinds of fat).

Saturated fats are the bad fat guys in the food gang. These are the artery clogging agents that put your kid at risk of heart disease and other illnesses. Three cookies, for instance, have 8 grams of fat, 2.5 grams of which are saturated fats. That means that nearly half of all its fat comes from saturated fats. The rice cakes, by contrast, contain no fats or saturated fats.

In general, try to avoid foods that are high in saturated fats. No more than 10 percent of all fat calories should come from saturated fats. For example, someone on a 2,000-calorie diet should consume no more than 20 grams of saturated fats a day.

Canning Cholesterol

High cholesterol levels increase the risk for heart disease. Adults and kids over two should eat less than 300 milligrams of dietary cholesterol per day. (Cholesterol content is measured in milligrams, not grams.) Remember, cholesterol comes mostly from animal sources, and organ meats are also high in cholesterol. So don't let your kids binge on red meats, eggs, and other cholesterol-rich foods.

Looking back at the cookie comparison, neither the rice cakes nor the cookies have any cholesterol.

Skipping Sodium

"Please pass the salt," your kids plead in unison. Think twice about it. *Sodium*, the component of salt, is responsible for water retention and high blood pressure in salt-sensitive people. Children ages 7 to 10 should keep sodium intake between 600 and 1800 milligrams. Kids who are 11 or older can increase their intake to the 900 to 2700 milligrams range.

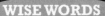

Sodium is a trace mineral that helps keep your body fluid in balance—but too much can be harmful to your health. Sodium is found in salt and processed food.

Warning: Sodium adds up quickly. Three ounces of tuna, for instance, has 303 milligrams of sodium. The same amount of salami has 1,922 milligrams of the stuff. Most foods are not considered high in sodium unless they have over 300 mg. per serving. Foods with less than 140 mg. are low-sodium; foods with 140-300 are "moderate." Fresh fruit is naturally low in sodium.

Calculating Carbohydrates

The Total Carbohydrates item has two subcategories: *dietary fiber* and *sugar*. Fiber can help lower cholesterol and reduce the risk of certain diseases. Try to choose foods with at least three grams of dietary fiber per serving, aiming anywhere between 25 and 35 grams a day.

Some simple sugars (like soda pop) are literally "empty calories" because they contain calories but no nutrients. Try to avoid these. But other simple sugars (like those found in milk and fruit) are full of nutrients. One cup of milk, for instance, has 12 grams of carbohydrates, 11 grams of sugar, and no fiber. But it's also full of protein and calcium. Simple sugar found in fruits is also full of nutrients. So the basic advice: It's OK for kids to get simple sugars from fruit sources and milk, but not from junk food.

Let's look at our comparison: One serving of the chocolate chip cookie, for instance, has 21 grams of carbohydrates, 10 grams of it from sugar. The rice cake, on the other hand, has 8 grams of carbohydrates, which has 0 grams of sugar.

To figure out how much complex carbohydrate each serving of food contains (remember, at least half of your child's diet should consist of carbohydrates), look at the label to see how much simple sugar is in one serving of the product. Then subtract that amount from the number of total carbohydrates to find out how much complex carbohydrate a serving of the product contains.

Piling on the Protein

Kids (and adults) need .36 grams of protein per pound of body weight daily. Most people eat way more than that amount. The best animal protein sources come from beef, poultry, eggs, and fish. But beware: These sources of protein are also high in cholesterol and fat.

The chocolate chip cookies have 2 grams of protein per serving and the rice cakes have one.

MOM KNOWS BEST

Although meats don't have to carry nutrition labels, look for nutrition facts posters in the meat department or ask your grocer for nutritional information.

DAILY VALUES: VALUE ADDED INFORMATION

Wait, the fun isn't over yet. It's time to translate all these calorie counts and fat grams into percentages. You're probably thinking, Why add insult to injury, right? Wrong.

Believe it or not, the Percent Daily Value will make your life easier. Instead of counting how many grams of fat and other nutrients your child eats, you can just look at the Percent Daily Value, which indicates how much of a day's recommended amount of each nutrient your child gets in a single serving. Keep in mind that these percentages are based on a 2,000 calorie diet.

Take, for example, one eight-ounce serving of freshly squeezed orange juice. Total carbohydrates: 25 g, or eight percent of Daily Value—which means that the OJ contains eight percent of the total carbohydrates your child needs for the day. The serving also contains 250 percent Daily Value for vitamin C—more than twice the amount he needs every day.

In addition to saving you time, the Percent Daily Value also helps you from falling into the trap of thinking that high numbers next to certain nutrients are bad, and low numbers are good.

You might think that a food with 140 milligrams of sodium, for instance, is high in sodium because 140 sounds like large number.

In reality, that amount represents less than six percent of the daily value for sodium (which is 2,400 for adults).

Follow this guideline: For total fat, saturated fat, cholesterol, and sodium, choose foods with a low Percent Daily Value. You want a higher Percent Daily Value for carbohydrates, dietary fiber, and all vitamins and minerals.

ALL IN THE FAMILY

Federal regulators require that most ingredients used in making a product be listed on the food label. Ingredients are listed in decreasing order by weight. One frozen chicken pot pie, for instance, lists these ingredients: pie filling, chicken broth, cooked diced chicken, potatoes, carrots, peas, and seasonings. If you want a pie with lots of peas, you better look for another brand. The peas are at the bottom of the line.

Daily Values for Nutritional Items Based on a 2,000 Calorie Diet

FOOD COMPONENT	DAILY VALUE (BASED ON 2,000-CALORIE DIET)
Total fat	65 grams
Saturated fat	20 grams
Cholesterol	300 grams
Sodium	2,400 milligrams
Potassium	3,500 milligrams
Total carbohydrate	300 grams
Dietary fiber	25 grams
Protein	50 grams
Vitamin A	5,000 international units
Vitamin C	60 milligrams
Calcium	1,000 milligrams
Iron	18 milligrams
Vitamin D	400 international units
Vitamin E	30 international units

FOOD COMPONENT	DAILY VALUE (BASED ON 2,000-CALORIE DIET)
Vitamin K	80 micrograms
Thiamin	1.5 milligrams
Riboflavin	1.7 milligrams
Niacin	20 milligrams
Vitamin B-6	2.0 milligrams
Folate	400 micrograms
Vitamin B-12	6.0 micrograms
Biotin	3 milligrams
Pantothenic acid	10 milligrams
Phosphorous	1000 milligrams
Iodine	150 micrograms
Magnesium	400 milligrams
Zinc	15 milligrams
Copper	2.0 milligrams
Selenium	70 micrograms
Manganese	2.0 milligrams
Chromium	120 micrograms
Molybdenum	75 micrograms
Chloride	3,400 milligrams

Source: Title 21 "Code of Federal Regulations," Parts 100-169, April 1, 1995, Section 101.9

MARKETING PLOYS

Without time to browse and little label know-how, many of us just grab items off the shelf that boast *low-fat*, *low-cholesterol*, and other benefits. A bag of cookies that claims *no cholesterol* may catch your eye and make its way into your basket. So might a cereal that features *100 percent* on the package, meaning that the cereal contains all of the USDA requirements for certain essential vitamins and minerals.

But what food manufacturers don't advertise (and when you think about it, why would they) is that those fabulous cookies are also high in saturated fats. The cereal may be high in sodium and sugar. Reading labels helps you evaluate the various nutritional claims made on the packages by manufacturers.

EVERYTHING YO'U NEED TO KNOW ABOUT NUTRITION CLAIMS

New nutrition laws spell out what terms manufacturers may use to describe the level of a nutrient in a food. Here are the guidelines spelled out by the FDA:

◆ **Free**   This term means that a product contains virtually no fat, saturated fat, cholesterol, sodium, sugars, or calories. For instance, *calorie-free* means the product has less than five calories per serving. *Sugar-free* and *fat-free* both mean that the product has less than .5 grams of the nutrient per serving.

◆ **Low**   This term is used for foods with small amounts of fat, saturated fat, cholesterol, sodium, or calories. Synonyms for low include *little*, *few*, and *low source of*.

  Low-fat means 3 grams or less per serving.

  Low saturated fat means 1 gram or less per serving.

  Low-sodium means 140 milligrams or less per serving.

  Very low-sodium means 35 milligrams or less per serving.

  Low-cholesterol means 20 milligrams or less and 2 grams or less of saturated fat per serving.

  Low-calorie means 40 calories or less per serving.

◆ **Lean and extra lean**   These terms describe the fat content of meat, poultry, and seafood. *Lean* means less than 10 grams of fat, 4.5 grams or less of saturated fat, and less than 95 milligrams of cholesterol per serving and per 100 grams.

  Extra lean means less than 5 grams of fat, less than 2 grams of saturated fat, and less than 95 milligrams of cholesterol per serving and per 100 grams.

◆ **High**   This term can be used if one serving of a food contains 20 percent or more of the Daily Value for a particular nutrient.

◆ **Good source**   This term means that one serving of a food contains 10 to 19 percent of the Daily Value for a particular nutrient.

◆ **Reduced**   This term means that a nutritionally altered product contains at least 25 percent less of a nutrient or of calories than the regular, or reference, product.

◆ **Less**   This term means that a food, whether altered or not, contains 25 percent less of a nutrient or of calories than the reference food. For instance, pretzels can be advertised as having 25 percent less fat than potato chips. *Fewer* is an acceptable synonym for *less*.

◆ **Light**   *Light* can either mean that a nutritionally altered product has one-third fewer calories or half the fat of the reference food. If the food gets 50 percent or more of its calories from fat, the reduction must be 50 percent of the fat. *Light* can also be used if the sodium content of a low-calorie, low-fat food has been reduced by 50 percent. One tablespoon of Kraft regular mayo, for instance, has 11 grams of fat and 100 calories. Light mayo, on the other hand, has 5 grams of fat and only 50 calories.

◆ **More**   This term means that a serving of food, whether altered or not, contains a nutrient that is at least 10 percent of the Daily Value more than the reference food. The 10 percent of Daily Value requirement also applies to *fortified*, *enriched*, and *added* claims, but the food must be altered in those cases. Take, for example, Rice Dream Vanilla. The regular drink has no vitamin A, D, and only two percent calcium. The Enriched with A&D plus Calcium has 10 percent vitamin A, 25 percent vitamin D, and 30 percent calcium.

The law also spells out definitions for *fresh*, *healthy*, and other health claims in food. Although these definitions can help you pick products that meet your child's nutritional needs, the best strategy is to read the nutrition label and take packaging claims with a grain of salt (or low-sodium salt substitute).

THE LEAST YOU NEED TO KNOW

♦ Nutritional information on the label is designed for the average American who takes in about 2,000 calories a day—and based on a diet made up of less than 30 percent fat, 15 percent protein, 55 percent carbohydrates, and less than 300 milligrams of cholesterol.

♦ Teenagers need between 2,200 and 2,800 calories a day (preteens need slightly less).

♦ Choose foods that have a big difference between the total number of calories and the number of fat calories. The larger the difference, the less fat.

♦ For total fat, saturated fat, cholesterol, and sodium, choose foods with a low Percent Daily Value. You want a higher Percent Daily Value for carbohydrates, dietary fiber, and all vitamins and minerals.

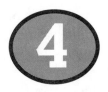

Buy the Right Stuff

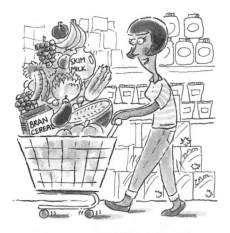

Now that you've achieved label literacy, put all that knowledge to good use and fill up your shopping cart with food that's good for your kids and tasty too (don't forget that part!). Strolling down the aisle can be fun (or at least productive) when you know what your children should eat and how to check the labels to ensure you are buying the right stuff.

DINNER DILEMMAS

Scenario 1: Your child says, "Mom, I'm hungry," and opens the refrigerator door. A precariously balanced box of chocolate dough-nuts falls off the top shelf and into your kid's hands. "Not before dinner," you warn and then check your cupboard for something

43

healthy to munch on. Your heart drops: Cinnamon Toast Crunch, a bag of potato chips, and Ritz crackers—all of them full of sugar and fat.

Scenario 2: You just got home from work and begin the ritual of "What shall we have tonight?" You find leftover chicken in the fridge, but not enough to feed the family. You forgot to thaw out the brisket and have your babysitter put it in the oven. All you've got for vegetables is spinach, and you are way too tired to fight with your kids over eating that. And to be fair, did you like spinach as a kid? The result: everyone piles in the car to go get a bite.

The dinner dilemma takes place in one way or another in many American homes, but you can lessen the turmoil if you are more organized about food shopping and making meals. Keeping the refrigerator and pantry stocked with healthful foods is your and your partner's job.

AVOID SHOPPING DISTRESS

Should the kids come along for the shopping field trip? This question is a tricky one. If you are like most moms, you probably have no time to shop during the day, so you pick up your kids from school and drag them down the supermarket aisles.

The advantages to taking your kids shopping with you are that you can introduce them to good foods and get them to help pick out their favorite fruits and vegetables, but timing is everything. If you go shopping after work, and your child is crabby, be prepared to leave behind a cart full of food and stomp out of the store. And then, what alternative do you have but going out to eat?

Everyone has different schedules. One mother goes shopping after her children go to bed to avoid fights she knows will arise if the kids go with her. She can browse over the display counter, compare products for price and nutrition, and enjoy the package designs. Another mom shops on Sunday afternoon while her husband spends quality time with the kids. My only warning: Don't go food shopping right after work when the market is swarming with tired workers like yourself who won't let you get in line ahead of them even if your child is incessantly kicking the magazine rack and indiscriminately throwing candy into the cart.

Here are some supermarket survival tips:

♦ Don't take hungry or worn-out kids with you. They'll kvetch and drive you crazy.

♦ When the rested, refreshed kids do come along, let them pick out their favorite fruits and vegetables.

♦ Send kids on a mission to retrieve certain items for you.

♦ Let your kids know ahead of time what they can or can't buy to avoid fights over what goes into the cart.

MAKE A LIST, CHECK IT TWICE

You can shop at chain supermarkets or healthy food stores. Lots of supermarkets carry healthful foods because of consumer demand. Some of them have aisles specializing in items that are low-calorie, low-sodium, low-cholesterol, and low-fat. On many shelves, low-fat versions of foods are next to the originals. Chain health food stores are popping up everywhere. There you can find substitutes for hot dogs and hamburgers as well as whole-wheat burritos and other specialties. Your child may enjoy these stores because they have hip displays and are different from the typical health food stores (usually perceived by kids to have rows and rows of pills, boring looking cookies, and a strange smell).

The first step before you walk out the door to the grocery store is to make a shopping list. The list is the key to being organized. Don't skip the list! If you do, you'll end up buying products you already have (like ketchup, salad dressings, and potatoes) and forgetting the items you need (like hamburger meat to go with the Hamburger Helper you just threw in the cart). When you are shopping, you can easily go on autopilot and just yank items off the shelf. A list keeps you focused.

You can approach food shopping in various ways. One way is to make your list in whatever order you want and just check off the items you've picked up as you go aisle by aisle. Many of us shop this way, but it isn't the most efficient method, because you waste a lot of time looking over the list. A better way is to think about the layout of your supermarket and then put together a list based on your usual travel path.

If the Food Pyramid makes it easier for you to determine what your child needs, make a list of each food group and write down what you want to buy under each category. Make sure you know where everything is in the supermarket, so you just have to go down each aisle once. Otherwise you'll be hopping around the store, and it won't be fun, especially on high heels.

Author Susan Price also suggests that you check to see whether your supermarket offers delivery services so you can order what you want by phone or fax. You'll probably have to pay a delivery fee, but it's worth it if you'd rather spend time with your kids at home than haul everyone up and down aisles. If your kid wants to come along for the nutritional education, take her when the stores are less crowded and when you are up to it. Other possibilities are to give your babysitter a shopping list or pay a high school helper to go to the store for you.

MOM KNOWS BEST

You'll want to buy certain items regardless of nutritional value. But if you want to buy certain low-fat, low-cholesterol products, put a sign next to them on the list so you don't forget. If your child needs more fiber, for instance, the mark next to bread will remind you to choose a high-fiber loaf.

ALL THE VEGGIES YOU CAN EAT

Most veggies are low in calories and are excellent sources of essential nutrients, such as fiber, vitamins A and C, potassium, calcium, and iron. Buy different vegetables every week because your children are bound to get all the minerals and vitamins they need from them.

MOM KNOWS BEST

Darker veggies tend to be more nutritional. Pale, small carrots have far less vitamin A than mature, bright-orange carrots. Dark-green leafy vegetables, like spinach and leaf lettuce, are better than light green, iceberg lettuce. Don't buy vegetables that have sat around in the bin for a couple of days; they may be cheaper, but they've lost their levels of vitamins A and C. How can you tell that the veggies are fresh? That's easy. They don't look rotten or bruised up—like the decaying vegetables in your fridge that you've forgotten about.

Fresh vegetables are the best. The more color they have, the more vitamins and minerals they contain. Many veggies are available year-round, and some come already washed and cut so all you have to do when you get home is open the bag and eat them raw or quickly pop them into the microwave or steamer pot. You can then serve them with or without dressing.

One mom I know buys a five-pound bag of small, unpeeled carrots and keeps them in the refrigerator for a couple of weeks. She just places a bowl of carrots on the table before dinner as a healthy snack. When the carrots are there, kids will eat them, especially if Mom puts a moratorium on junk food, at least for that hour before dinner.

For a complete and balanced diet, your kids need to eat many different kinds of vegetables. Here is what different veggies have to offer:

◆ Broccoli has calcium, potassium, iron, fiber, vitamin A, vitamin C, folic acid, and niacin.

◆ Carrots provide vitamin A, potassium, and fiber.

◆ Corn provides vitamin A, potassium, and fiber.

◆ Lettuce (iceberg, romaine, and other varieties) provides vitamin C and folic acid.

◆ Mushrooms provide potassium, niacin, and riboflavin.

◆ Green peas provide vitamin A, folic acid, potassium, protein, and fiber.

◆ Potatoes provide potassium, most B vitamins, vitamin C, protein, and fiber.

◆ Spinach provides vitamin A, folic acid, potassium, and fiber.

◆ Tomatoes provide vitamins A and C and potassium.

If you can't go shopping often, or if your green veggies frequently turn brown because you forgot they were there, consider buying frozen vegetables. They come in many combinations (cut, chopped, pureed), and the freezer keeps the nutrients locked in. Canned vegetables can also be good substitutes for fresh vegetables, because they provide almost the same nutritional value. However, many canned goods have high sodium levels, so try to buy cans that say *low in sodium.*

ALL IN THE FAMILY

If you don't know what to cook with vegetables and hate skimming through cookbooks, look into cooking software programs. You can punch in what you've got, and the computer spews out what you can do with it. Some programs can even help you make shopping lists or calculate measurements so you can change the number of servings a recipe makes.

A FEAST OF FRUITS

Throw as many fruits as you want into your cart—your children are supposed to eat two to four servings a day. Fruits are low in calories and sodium, high in carbohydrates and fiber, and a good source of vitamins A and C and potassium. Because vitamin C enhances the absorption of iron, eating fruit can also boost the benefits of iron intake from other foods.

Buy fresh fruit weekly, if not more often, because if you keep it around much longer, it starts to rot. (Look under your fruit bowl; you are bound to find a wrinkled, crumpled pear half its original size.) Be sure that your kids eat the fruits rich in vitamins A and C right away because those vitamins are easily destroyed. If the selection of fruits like bananas, pears, peaches, and plums are not ripe, leave them outside your refrigerator to soften, but this time try to remember they are there.

Buy in-season fruits; they'll probably be juicier and cheaper. If your child is dying for peaches in the middle of winter, then buy canned fruits, but go with the ones labeled *no added sugar* or *unsweetened*. The heavy syrups in canned fruit are filled with calories and sugar.

Will jams and jellies do when your child refuses to eat fruit? I think not. By law, jelly, jam, or preserves must be sweetened with sugar and must contain 55 percent sugar by weight. When fruit juice is used as a sweetener, the product has to be called a "spread" or "conserve." But whatever you call them, they both have about the same amount of sugar and calories. So, let them eat apples.

Put juice containers in your cart, but push your kids to eat real fruit instead. Resist buying the more kid-friendly, sugar-flavored drinks or cocktails. Stick to drinks that are labeled 100 percent juice.

Here is what's in the fruits your child likes to eat:

◆ Apples contain potassium and fiber.

◆ Bananas provide lots of potassium and some vitamin A and fiber.

◆ Cantaloupes provide vitamins A and C and potassium.

◆ Oranges provide lots of vitamin C, potassium, and folic acid.

◆ Strawberries provide vitamin C, along with potassium, folic acid, and fiber.

◆ Watermelon provides vitamin A and some vitamin C.

◆ Grapes provide some fiber.

Getting your child into the habit of grabbing an apple or a carrot stick whenever she wants a snack will help her develop healthful eating patterns that will hopefully last for the rest of her life. Most supermarkets have a wide selection of fresh, luscious produce, so you could mix and match fruits, combine veggies in unusual ways, or just order healthful carry-out!

STARCH: WHERE IT'S AT

Children of all ages love cereal, breads, grains and pasta, so you're in luck in this category. Nutrition experts suggest that grain-based foods make up at least half of our calories—so let your child fill up on complex carbohydrates!

Breaking Bread

White bread, which has little fiber, is still the most popular brand purchased. Whole-grain breads have more vitamins, minerals, and calories than white bread, and they also have fiber. Before you pitch any loaves into your cart, check the label to make sure your brand is rich in fiber. If the bread contains two or more grams of fiber per slice, it's a keeper.

When you're buying breads, pitas, bagels, or crackers, stick with whole-wheat, multigrain, rye, millet, oat bran, oat, and cracked-wheat varieties. (Beware: *Wheat* bread may sound just as good as *whole-wheat*, but wheat bread is just a mix of white and whole-wheat flour. For a product to be called *whole-wheat*, it has to be made from 100 percent whole-wheat flour.)

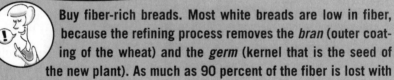

MOM ALWAYS SAID

Buy fiber-rich breads. Most white breads are low in fiber, because the refining process removes the *bran* (outer coating of the wheat) and the *germ* (kernel that is the seed of the new plant). As much as 90 percent of the fiber is lost with the removal of the germ and the bran.

Cereal Madness

If your kids have been begging you to come shopping, this aisle most likely is the reason why. They are dazzled by the irresistible boxes showing their favorite sports figures or cartoon characters.

Manufacturers cater to kids' whims, and we, the parents, have to deal with the fallout—the avalanche of cereal boxes that topple into our cart as we walk down this aisle. When you buy cereal, put your foot down. Check the label, because many cereals are made almost entirely of sugar. Your kid may as well be eating a bowl of candy.

General Mill's Wheaties, for instance, has 3 grams of dietary fiber and 4 grams of sugar. Compare that to Kellogg's Apple Jacks, which has 1 gram of fiber and 13 grams of sugar. A serving of Wheaties is 110 calories. Apple Jacks has slightly fewer calories at 100 per serving, but Wheaties has more vitamin A, vitamin C, iron, zinc, and other minerals and vitamins. They both have the same amount of carbohydrate (24 mg), but one is obviously higher in nutrition than the other.

Choose cereals that have at least 2 grams of fiber per serving. Go for cereals with *bran* in their name, such as Bran Flakes and Raisin Bran. Best choices are cereals made with whole-grain puffed wheat and corn or whole-grain wheat, oat, or rice flakes. Don't forget to throw in some hot cereals. Stick with unsweetened varieties of oatmeal, grits, cream of rice, and cream of wheat. Sweeten them up with fresh fruit.

Lotsa Pasta—and Rice, Too!

Cram lots and lots of pasta and rice into your cart. Your kids love them, the price is right, and they're rich in complex carbohydrate and protein. Pasta made from whole grains contains fiber as well. You can buy pasta and rice in bulk.

Younger kids love all the twirls and shapes of pastas. Experts suggest that you serve pastas in dinosaur shapes, in smiley faces, or decorated in ways that catch your kid's imagination. But if you play that trick on teens, all you're gonna catch is flack. These guys are straight shooters when it comes to food and serving anything cutesy will be viewed with suspicion and scorn.

MILK THAT COW, BUT TRIM THE FAT

Milk products are excellent sources of protein, calcium, some B vitamins, and vitamin A. Most milk is also fortified with vitamin D. According to the government, milk and milk products account for more than 75 percent of the calcium available in our food supply. Calcium intake is considered to be one of the major factors in the prevention of osteoporosis (the loss of bone mass that most commonly afflicts postmenopausal women). Children ages 6 to 10 need about 800 to 1,200 milligrams of calcium a day. Adolescents and young adults ages 11 to 24 need between 1,200 to 1,500 milligrams a day. One cup of low-fat milk (one percent fat) contains 300 milligrams of calcium.

Buy low-fat or skim versions of all dairy products, because many regular dairy products are high in saturated fats, a problem for those concerned with cholesterol levels. Check the labels on low-fat and skim milk to be sure that they have been fortified with vitamins A and D. Sometimes these fat-soluble vitamins are lost in the defatting process. If you can't stand the thought of eating some of the fat-free cheeses because they taste like rubber, try the low-fat ones, which contain three to five grams of fat per ounce.

MOM KNOWS BEST

 Some tips from experts: Select a milk carton from the bottom of the dairy case; those on top may not be getting cooled property. Pick up the milk right before you pay to lessen the time it's out of the refrigerator. Always, always check the *sell by* date on the carton.

POTENT PROTEINS

As you remember from the previous chapter, protein is key to our children's well-being. They can get protein from animal products like meat, fish, poultry, eggs, milk, and cheese. Or, they can combine incomplete protein sources to make up the whole chain of amino acids. Meat and poultry are among the highest quality sources of protein around.

Poultry is leaner than beef, especially if the skin is removed before cooking. Some people like to cook with the skin on to retain the moistness. No problem; just remove the skin before you serve it to your child. Your leanest poultry choices:

◆ skinless chicken breast

◆ turkey breast (white meat, no skin)

◆ Cornish hen (no skin)

Serve your children less duck, fried chicken, or chicken nuggets—all of which are high in fat and cholesterol. Instead of giving your kids chicken nuggets, for example, try giving them grilled chicken tenders. A chicken breast without the skin has only 131 calories, 6 grams of fat, and 64 milligrams of dietary cholesterol. Chicken nuggets, by comparison, have 180 calories and 9 grams of fat.

Certain cuts of meat are very high in fat. Before you throw meat in your cart, look for visible fat and *marbling*, which refers to the presence of white, rubbery, vein-like streaks that run throughout the meat. Also look at the grades assigned to meat cuts at the slaughterhouse:

◆ *Prime* usually has the most fat but is the most tender.

◆ *Choice* is moderately fatty and tender.

◆ *Select* means lean.

The leanest meats (fat trimmed) include:

◆ Three-oz. sirloin tip roast, 156 calories, 33 percent fat, 69 mg. of cholesterol.

◆ Three-oz. top loin steak, 163 calories, 36 percent fat, 65 mg. of cholesterol

◆ Three-oz. ground chuck, 240 calories, 57 percent fat, 87 mg. of cholesterol

◆ Three-oz. veal chop, loin cut, 192 calories, 36 percent fat 135 mg. of cholesterol

Excellent Eggs

Eggs are a great source of protein, vitamin A, and other micronutrients. But they are also high in cholesterol; one egg has about 213 milligrams, more than half the limit recommended for one day. (The cholesterol is all located in the egg yolk. You can use the whites for cooking without adding cholesterol.) The key in egg consumption is moderation. Look at what else your child is eating during the day, and then decide whether an egg would add to her nutrition.

MOM KNOWS BEST

Don't buy egg cartons that have been sitting in the supermarket aisle waiting to be shelved. Eggs can easily spoil if not refrigerated. Also, open the egg carton to make sure none of the eggs are cracked, and try not to crack one when you are checking. If one egg is cracked, get a new box.

If your child can't have eggs at all because of allergies, buy the egg-free substitutes located either in the frozen-food section or the dairy section.

Shell Out Fish

You'll know you are getting to the fish section because of the seaweed smell, the wet floor, and the guy in the back holding a hose. If you are with kids, you won't be able to even peek at the counter because your children will be gagging. Kids rarely like fish, but some kids love the fish counter—not as food, but as an exhibit of sea life. If you have one like that, this is the time to teach him about which fish is more nutritious to eat.

One kid-friendly fish is tuna, which generally comes out of a can, with few signs of its origins. Buy tuna packed in water, not oil. A three-and-a-half ounce serving of oil-packed tuna has about 300 calories and 20 grams of fat. Packed with water, the same amount of tuna has 131 calories and only a half a gram of fat.

Lean fish choices include cod, flounder, haddock, monkfish, sea bass, tuna, halibut, mullet, red snapper, and swordfish. Fattier fish include salmon, albacore tuna, mackerel, and herring. But don't stop buying salmon if your teen is into it, since most fattier fish have polyunsaturated fats—the "good for you" fat that fights against heart disease.

Get a Leg Up on Legumes

What the heck are legumes? They're a special group of vegetables that includes dried beans, peas, lentils, and bean curd (tofu). These foods supply protein, iron, zinc, magnesium, and B vitamins, and they are an excellent substitute for meat. But children can't live by legumes alone. These proteins are considered incomplete (as Chapter 2 explained, an incomplete protein doesn't have all the amino acids in tow), so you must supplement them with foods like rice, whole grains, nuts, and seeds.

About tofu: Your kids won't know what it is or where it is. Tofu is one of the highest protein vegetable foods, and it's low in calories. Tofu has no taste of its own, so it picks up the flavor of the ingredients with which it is mixed, making it ideal for soups, casseroles, dips, and salads. Some kids will eat tofu without realizing it; others will immediately suspect that you sneaked something in.

Look for legumes with bright colors; kids hate eating foods that don't look nice, even if they are nutritional. You can use black beans, for instance, to make soups or stews or to have as a main course along with rice and a salad.

FREEZE AND EAT

Don't grimace when I suggest that you buy frozen meals to give your kids. Get off the guilt trip and on the wagon. Many frozen dinners are healthy and tasty. When you choose frozen meals, pick out those that contain less than 400 total calories, 15 grams of fat, and 800 milligrams of sodium. Experts suggest that some frozen meals are low in vitamins A and C and calcium. So if you serve these meals, consider either adding a cup of skim milk, two cups of broccoli (although that may be too much for your child), or other items to make up for the deficiency.

In addition to buying frozen prepared meals, you can freeze some ingredients to maintain their freshness until you are ready to use them. You can freeze uncooked meats, poultry, fish, soup stocks, prepared and precooked dishes, hard cheeses, milk, butter, egg whites and yolks, chopped herbs, many fruits and vegetables, cooked grains, and pastry shells. If you freeze fruits, throw them in the freezer right after you buy them to make sure that they retain their vitamins. Meats and poultry have to be repackaged tightly if you want to freeze them.

Do not freeze foods with high water content (such as salads, cucumbers, cantaloupes, and potatoes), dairy products (such as cream-based sauces, yogurt, and mayonnaise), salad dressings, fried foods, or hard-boiled eggs.

SPICE UP YOUR MEALS

Doesn't anybody eat anything plain anymore? Many people do, but you can't tell from the looks of the condiment aisle. This section is full of products that could turn your dull meals into delicious ones. But be careful; some condiments have a lot of fat, calories, or sodium. A tablespoon of tartar sauce, for example, adds 70 calories, almost all of them from fat. Plain mayonnaise has 99 calories a spoonful and is almost 100 percent fat.

Don't give up condiments, but eat them sparingly. Make sure the following are stocked in your cupboard:

◆ Ketchup

◆ Salsa

◆ Mustard

◆ Barbecue sauce

◆ Fat-free ranch dressing

◆ Teriyaki sauce, low sodium

◆ Worcestershire sauce

◆ Balsamic vinegar

◆ Cider vinegar

Kids are always asking for more salt. Most fast foods and canned foods contain plenty of salt, but your kids may not need as much salt if your food is tastier (don't take offense; I'm no gourmet cook, either). Buy salt-free spices to put some zest into your meals.

You can use many of these spices in ethnic dishes, so you can widen your children's palate:

- ◆ Cajun spices
- ◆ Garlic powder
- ◆ Curry
- ◆ Mexican seasonings
- ◆ Italian seasonings

What oil should you buy? Stick to unsaturated oils. They include, in part:

- ◆ Vegetable oil
- ◆ Olive oil
- ◆ Peanut oil
- ◆ Canola oil
- ◆ Soybean oil
- ◆ Nonstick cooking sprays
- ◆ Corn oil
- ◆ Safflower oil
- ◆ Sunflower oil

The whole point of buying the right stuff is to make sure you have all the foods you need within arm's reach at home, so when everyone announces they're starved, you can quickly whip up something nutritious. The *Working Parents Help Book*, (1996, Peterson's, Susan Crites Price and Tom Price), suggests additional convenience items you should pick up from the grocery store:

- ◆ Garlic, minced and packed with water in jars
- ◆ Cut-up vegetables from the salad bar
- ◆ Bags of shredded (low-fat) cheese, which you can freeze for long storage
- ◆ Canned chicken and beef broth

◆ Frozen waffles and bagels for quick kid snacks and breakfasts

◆ Seasoned bread crumbs

◆ Flat bread, for individual child-size pizzas and appetizers

◆ Frozen bread dough

◆ Refrigerated cookie dough

◆ Frozen mashed potatoes (they taste better than instant and also can be used to thicken soups)

◆ Varieties of canned, cooked beans for use in soups, casseroles, and chili

THE LEAST YOU NEED TO KNOW

◆ To stock your kitchen with healthy foods, find out what you've already got and what your children need to eat to stay in good shape and develop well-balanced eating habits.

◆ Before you dash out to the market, make a shopping list.

◆ Throw lots of fruits and veggies into your cart, but not too much because these items lose vitamins if not eaten right away.

◆ Buy low-fat dairy products when possible, and stick to lower fat meats like chicken and turkey.

◆ Zero in on grains made with whole-grain flour. Choose cereals that have at least two grams of fiber per serving and are low in sugar.

◆ Flavor your foods with low-fat condiments and spices.

5

Cooking Tips and Shortcuts for Busy Moms

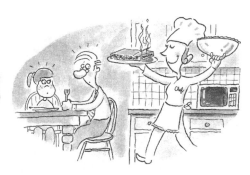

Your kitchen is now stocked with healthy foods. Your fridge glows with color: red juicy apples, green leafy lettuce, yummy yellow peppers, bright orange, um, oranges. Your cupboard overflows with brown rice, couscous, fiber-filled crackers, and other nutrient-rich foods. Now the question is: How do you get your kids to eat them?

My suggestion: Plan dinner ahead of time. It's hard to think about what to make for dinner when you've just gotten home from work, your kid is tugging at you to play UNO, and the phone is ringing off the hook. How many times have you looked in your refrigerator and decided you just couldn't make any more decisions that day? In this chapter, you'll learn how to make quick, easy, balanced meals. You'll also learn how to revamp your family's favorites with a few substitutions to increase the nutritional value of your menus or add servings—rather than substitutes—to meals. Such additions could be serving two veggies instead of one.

COOKING GADGETS

Before you venture into the wonderful world of fast, nutritious home-cooking, you have to make sure your kitchen is properly equipped. Walking into a store to buy kitchen utensils can be overwhelming. Hundreds of cooking gadgets dangle above you, some of which you've gotten as wedding gifts and never used and others that look so strange you can't imagine ever using them.

You don't have to get fancy. For quick, easy cooking you just need the following equipment:

- **Microwaves make magic.** Can you imagine life without a microwave? I can't. You can use a microwave to cook, heat, thaw, and bake. You don't have to use butter or oil because the microwave uses moist heat to cook your food. The fast cooking doesn't give nutrients a chance to escape, so your food retains all the vitamins and minerals.

- **Woks work wonders.** A wok is one of the most useful pieces of cooking equipment you'll ever have. With a wok, the food cooks fast, and you only have to use a drop of oil. Like a microwave, the wok cooks food without destroying its nutrients.

- **Veggies stay green in a steamer.** Avoid dunking vegetables into boiling water. The water drowns out a lot of the nutrients. A vegetable steamer is a metal insert placed inside cooking pots that holds vegetables above the boiling water. Just cover the pot and within minutes the veggies are done!

- **Food processors do the daily grind.** If you plan to substitute fats and oils with vegetables, you need a food processor. Processors come with many options, including slicing, shredding, and chopping, and are ideal for making soups, vegetable purees, and side dishes.

- ◆ **Pop it in the toaster oven.** Don't underrate the importance of the old-fashioned toaster oven. Use it regularly to make toast, bagel pizzas, and heat up sandwiches.

- ◆ **Non-stick pans make non-fat meals.** Non-stick pans look like little woks. You can sauté meats and vegetables, fry eggs, and make other foods in non-stick pans with just a tad of oil. You can also spray non-stick spray on them and do away with the oil altogether.

ALL IN THE FAMILY

You want to cook low-fat foods? Forget about frying. Stick to steaming, stir-frying, broiling, grilling, barbecuing, and microwaving. Use as little saturated fat as possible, limit high cholesterol foods, cook less fatty red meats, use less salt, avoid excess sugar, cook with high-fiber products, and use low-fat dairy products.

MEAL OVERHAULS NOT NECESSARY

To cook healthy foods, you don't have to make radical changes. The last thing you should do is come home with a platter full of vegetables nobody recognizes and announce that sugar is dead. Your kids will rebel against the imposition, and you'll be pulling teeth to get them to take a bite. Remember: You want the kid to eat well, not go into shock.

You also don't have to be a gourmet cook to suit your children's palates. Most kids like less than a dozen foods, and they would be happy to eat them repeatedly. Most of what your kids like to eat can be made with low-fat, low-cholesterol ingredients, and your kids probably won't even know it. Modifying recipes isn't hard because most of the less-desirable substances in our foods come from just a few sources, namely fats (especially saturated fats).

Your child wants a chocolate shake? Use skim milk, fat-free frozen yogurt, and a dab of chocolate syrup. Your daughter is begging for french fries? No problem. Cut up a potato in strips, spray the strips with non-stick spray, toss in some spices, and bake them in the oven. Your children want fried chicken? Douse chicken breasts in egg substitute, roll them over bread crumbs, and bake them.

I urge friends to switch their kids into low-fat diets slowly. If your children drink whole milk, for example, start them on two percent, then switch to one percent, and finally switch to skim. It will take a while for your kids to lose the taste for fat. Or go from sugared cereals to cereals with less sugar and more fiber. Don't do it all at once; introduce the changes one at a time.

The following table shows substitutions for common cooking ingredients. When a recipe calls for one of the items on the left hand side, substitute with an item on the right column. Place the list somewhere in your kitchen so you can glance at it before you cook.

Easy Substitutes	
INSTEAD OF	*USE*
One egg	Two egg whites or $\frac{1}{4}$ cup of egg substitute
Cream	Canned evaporated skim milk
Whole milk	Skim milk
Sour cream	Nonfat yogurt or low-fat cottage cheese
Butter	Vegetable oil for cooking and baking
Cooking oil	Non-stick vegetable sprays, 1 or 2 tablespoons of defatted broth, water, wine, or pureed vegetables
Stick margarine	Soft tub margarine or imitation margarine
Mayonnaise	Reduced fat or fat-free mayonnaise
Cheese	Reduced fat or fat-free cheese

These substitutions will significantly lower the fat and cholesterol in your children's meals. You can also substitute veggie burgers for hamburgers and make spaghetti sauce with ground chicken or turkey rather than red meat. Remember: meatless products may have less fat than beef, but they aren't fat-free. When you do use meat, trim all the visible fat before you cook it.

Many kids won't pick up on the fact that you are serving healthful meals. To them, a sandwich is a sandwich, and besides, ketchup is a great taste equalizer.

POWERFUL PUREES

Unfortunately, not all healthy substitutions are quick. For example, some experts suggest that you replace olive oil in pasta sauces with baby carrot purees or mashed potatoes. It's a great idea! You can nix the oil and sneak veggies into your child's diet. But making purees is time-consuming. It isn't a thing you want to do when you come home from work with hungry eyes staring at you. Here's my advice: Puree the ingredients the night before (get your kids to help), and use the puree the next day or freeze it until you need it.

According to the ADA pamphlet *Skim The Fat: A Practical & Up To Date Food Guide* (1995), you can use vegetables as fat replacements for other items:

◆ Replace some of the fat in nut breads or cakes, like carrot cake or zucchini bread, with vegetable purees or juices

◆ Substitute pureed green peas for half the amount of mashed avocado in guacamole or other dips

◆ Replace fat in soups, sauces, muffins, or cakes with mashed yams or sweet potatoes

◆ Use potatoes to thicken lower-fat milks in cream soups and bisques

◆ Substitute a layer of vegetables in your favorite lasagna to replace meat or sausage

◆ Top your pizza with vegetables instead of meat

You also can puree fruit to use in baked goods. Traditionally, fats are used in these products to make them moist, but fruit can do the job just as well. If the original recipe calls for half a cup of fat, just add half a cup of pureed fruit instead.

The ADA pamphlet offers these additional tips:

◆ Dark-colored fruits, such as blueberries and prunes, are best used for dark-colored batters. You can add lighter-colored fruits, such as pears or applesauce, to almost any batter without changing its color.

- You can use pears and apples nearly universally in baking because their taste is very mild and unnoticeable. Apricots, prunes, and pineapple add a much stronger flavor. Bananas and peaches are somewhere in the middle, adding a little flavor, but never overwhelming.

- If you don't have a food processor to puree fruit, try using baby food. It is already pureed, has a very mild flavor, and is usually made without sugar.

TWO-MICROWAVE FAMILY

Whether you are heating up leftovers, making a meal from scratch, or thawing frozen food, you'll be standing in line waiting to use the microwave. This piece of equipment is truly a mom's best friend. You can cook dishes in a whiff, and there is less of a mess to clean up.

Microwaves are especially handy when everyone in the family is on a different meal schedule. For example, one mom I know makes a vegetable lasagna on nights when everyone does their own thing. When her son comes home from baseball practice, he heats up a bowl and eats it with bread and a salad (which she leaves in the refrigerator). This way, everyone eats a nutritious meal even though the family isn't eating together.

But microwaves can turn your food to mush or rubber if you don't know how to use them. *The Tufts University Guide to Total Nutrition* (Harper & Row Publishers, 1990) gives tips on how to make microwave magic work for you:

- Don't overcook. When foods are left in the microwave after the beep goes off, they can lose some of their nutrients because they are still technically cooking.

- Cover dishes to promote steaming. Covering dishes also accelerates cooking time.

- Cook small items only. Don't make huge briskets or turkey feasts in the microwave. These items won't cook well because they won't cook evenly.

◆ Use dishes that help food cook evenly. Don't throw in deep and narrow dishes; wide, shallow dishes work better. Round dishes are better than rectangular or square ones.

◆ Use the microwave to help you bake. Microwaves can cut preparation time even if you ultimately plan to bake the dish in the oven. Butter, margarine, and chocolate melt quickly and more evenly in the microwave than on a stove top.

◆ Re-wet when you reheat. Some dishes absorb all the liquid the first time they cook. So if you are serving leftovers, throw in a couple of tablespoons of water (avoid using butter).

◆ Cook food early and freeze it. Use your microwave to heat up leftovers or use it to cook foods for freezing. Don't worry about undercooking the food; the food will be fully cooked when you reheat it to serve.

◆ You don't have to brown meat over a frying pan in sizzling oil. Instead, brown it in the microwave. If you trim off the fat, more heat will get to the meat.

Your kids are now starting to use the microwave by themselves. To ensure safety, follow the American Academy of Pediatrics' recommendations:

◆ Make sure kids use pot holders when removing dishes from the microwave.

◆ Show older children how to open popcorn package containers so they don't burn their hands and faces with the steam.

◆ Teach kids to stir food well before tasting it to avoid uneven "hot spots."

KID-FRIENDLY RECIPES

Many children's recipe books offer great suggestions for making low-fat dishes, but many recipes you'll find are time-consuming and not designed with busy parents in mind. The American Heart Association, for instance, has a terrific recipe to make oven-fried rather than deep-fried chicken nuggets. But the equipment you need to pull it off would drive you nuts. You need a measuring cup, resealable plastic bag, rolling pin, saucepan or small microwave-safe bowl, wax paper, baking sheet, mixing spoons, and more. Chances are you can't even find the briefcase that you put down five minutes ago, never mind cooking equipment you hardly ever use.

By contrast, the following dishes can be made on the spot and incorporate many of the food groups your child needs to grow healthy and strong:

◆ Pasta dishes with low-fat sauces. Toss in some vegetables and chicken and your dinner is made.

◆ Burrito (fat-free, whole wheat) stuffed with chicken, ground turkey, or beans and rice. Serve shredded lettuce and tomatoes on the side. (You can use the same recipe for tacos or tortillas.)

◆ Pizza. Buy prepared crust and add vegetables (green peppers, onions, mushrooms, or whatever your kid eats). Top it off with low-fat cheeses.

◆ Barbecued chicken, corn on the cob, and mashed potatoes.

◆ Turkey burgers, peas, and oven-fried potatoes.

◆ Macaroni and cheese (low-fat cheese) and peas.

◆ Bean or chicken soup with a grilled cheese sandwich (spray non-stick spray on a non-stick pan and on both slices of bread, and then cook over medium heat).

◆ French toast (for dinner? why not?). Dip the bread into egg substitute and spray non-stick spray onto the hot non-stick pan.

Dinner preparations don't have to be a hassle in order to be nutritious. Feed your kids the right nutrients and you've done the job. And if it takes you only 15 minutes to prepare, feel glad about it—not guilty because you aren't slaving over a hot stove. After all, the less time spent in the kitchen, the more time you'll have to read stories with your kids or help them with homework. Who has time to be June Cleaver?

DOING TWO THINGS AT ONE TIME

You probably tell your children, "I can't do two things at once." But you can do a lot more than you think while you are getting dinner ready. The key is organization and focus.

Here is what one mom does to maximize the use of every minute: The race starts at 6 P.M. when she storms through the front door, tears her kids away from the TV, tells them to set the table, and heads to the kitchen to boil the water for pasta. While the water heats up, she hurries to her room, kicks off her pumps, changes clothes, and washes her face. When she comes back down, she chucks the pasta into the water. At the same time, she grabs a bag of washed, cut veggies and hurls them into a microwave dish, covers it, and nukes it for a couple of minutes. Everything is ready at once. She tosses the pasta and veggies and adds a low-fat sauce. Voilá! Dinner is served. If stir-fry is more your style, get the rice cooking while you are changing, and when you come back, throw the veggies in the wok. Toss the foods together and pour a low-fat, low-sodium stir-fry sauce over it.

Buying vegetables that are already washed and chopped saves you lots of time. But if you think these items are too costly, cut the veggies yourself, with your kids' help, the night before so they are ready to use when you need them.

For some ideas on low-fat, quick, and easy-to-fix healthy recipes, *Quick and Healthy Vols. I and II*, by Brenda Ponichtera, published by ScaleDown (503-296-5859), are terrific cookbooks with quick, easy to fix healthy recipes.

RECYCLING FOOD

Whatever you do, never throw food away that you could recycle for other meals. Ever gone to a hotel or vacation spot where every buffet was made up of food you'd seen elsewhere the day before? Prunes served in a bowl of dried fruits appeared in your omelet. Raw vegetables were thrown into a stir-fry dish with the same chicken you ate yesterday. Using leftovers to make meals is easy and quick.

One mom, for instance, always throws extra chicken on the grill so her kids can take chicken sandwiches to school the day after their barbecue. Two days later, the family has chicken tacos for dinner. By that point, her family is practically cackling, so she switches to spaghetti with ground turkey sauce (which, by the way, she made tons of so she could freeze a batch and eat it weeks later).

Soups are another great leftover idea. One mom makes huge vats of hearty soups on Sunday nights to serve for dinner as well as one other day during the week. Kids fill up their own bowls, grab a chunk of whole-wheat bread, and enjoy the meal. If your child hates soup, try emptying out the liquid and serving the vegetables on the side in a tortilla.

If this cooking style suits you, make sure you keep labels on frozen items. Your son will be disappointed if instead of having veggie burgers (which he thinks are hamburgers) for dinner, he has to eat lentil stew. Do you blame him?

GOOD MORNING FOOD

Breakfast is the most important meal to eat, yet it is also the one most frequently skipped. Studies have shown that kids who miss breakfast can't concentrate on their work and become restless by late morning. In the morning, your child should have foods that provide quick energy and those that release energy more slowly. Breakfasts should include a protein source, a bread or cereal, a fruit or vegetable, and a small amount of fat and milk.

What? All that and still be out by 7:30? All the experts say, "try to make breakfast fun." Fun? At 6 A.M. when your husband screams because the hot water ran out, when your teenager refuses to get up, and when you have an important meeting first thing in the morning? I don't think so. At that time, most of us just strive for bearable.

The easiest food to give your child in the morning is cereal with milk. It's best to serve cereals with high iron and fiber. If your kid wants something sweet, jazz up unsweetened cereal with sliced bananas, strawberries, or other fruit. You don't have to stick to the same old breakfast food, however. As long as the food is nutritious, the form doesn't matter.

MOM KNOWS BEST

Kids will often eat something if you sit with them for breakfast.

The AAP (American Academy of Pediatrics) suggests some alternative ideas for kids who don't want the typical breakfast:

- Breakfast shake: combine skim or one percent milk, fruit, and ice in a blender.

- Frozen banana: dip a banana in yogurt, and then roll it in crushed cereal. Freeze.

- Peanut butter spread on crackers, a tortilla, or apple slices.

- Leftover spaghetti, chicken, or pizza served hot or cold.

The biggest challenge for breakfast is getting teens out of bed. They'd rather sleep. If you can't shake your child awake, consider packing a breakfast for him to eat on the bus. You could give him a peanut butter or cheese sandwich, fruit, yogurt, or bran muffin. If you don't give him something, he may stop off at Dunkin' Donuts for a breakfast full of empty calories.

MOM KNOWS BEST

To get your kid to eat less-sugared cereal, serve sugar-free cereal with a little bit of her favorite sugar-loaded cereal on top. If she won't go for it, do half and half—her favorite sugared brand on top and the rest on the bottom. Then switch to putting sliced bananas, strawberries, raisins, and other naturally sweetened foods on top of the cereal. Adding fruit to the cereal increases the level of vitamin C and fiber.

THE LEAST YOU NEED TO KNOW

◆ To make quick meals, you need a microwave, wok, and other gadgets.

◆ Don't radically change the meals your kids love, just substitute lower-fat ingredients in your recipes.

◆ Avoid making rubbery food by learning how to use the microwave properly.

◆ Use leftovers in new meals.

◆ Make sure you send your kid off to school with a healthy breakfast.

6

I'm Not Eating THAT!

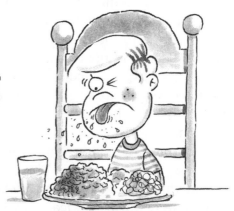

You've finally made your family a quick, healthful meal without much fuss. For dinner tonight, you're serving breaded chicken (a nugget look-alike of sorts), fresh corn, a cucumber and carrot salad, rolls, and watermelon. Everyone takes their seat around the table eager to eat—except your 9-year-old daughter, who's already scowling at the offerings.

Your heart sinks because she is the finicky child, the child who never likes anything you serve, won't try anything new, and whines a lot. She may be the joy of your life in other areas, but when it comes to eating, she is a drag. How do you deal with her? Should you force her to eat? The answer is no. This chapter will give you some insight about why your child may be finicky and what you can do to encourage her to try new foods to preserve her health—and your sanity.

AVOIDING FOOD FIGHTS

Most of us have a finicky child, or know one. Finicky children can be adventurous, fun-loving, interesting kids most of the time, but when it comes to food, they have a huge list of what they won't eat, don't like, and never want to try. And because eating is their least fun activity, they make everyone else suffer.

A typical scenario: The mother begs and pushes her daughter to eat something. When all else fails, mom dashes to the kitchen to cook a back-up. The dad, already agitated, takes his frustration out on the other kids, yelling at one for not sitting still and at the other for looking like a hoodlum. The mother gets mad at her husband for losing his cool. Who'd want to be at that table?

Yet family meals at least several times a week are crucial. During the time in children's lives when they are struggling for their independence, they need your support and reassurance. Forcing them to eat shuts doors to communication. Your children will resent you for interfering and being bossy and you'll be too busy picking at things that are wrong with them. The result is that your child won't hear his own internal voice to guide his actions, and he'll rely on you and others to tell him what to eat and how to act. This type of behavior can lead to food disorders.

It's just not worth fighting during dinner. Studies show that kids don't eat as well when they are constantly criticized by their parents on any topic. If you can't stop chastising your children, talk to a counselor to figure out why you react the way you do and to learn how to deal with your children better.

Parental Role in Children's Nutrition During Different Stages of Development	

School-age

CHARACTERISTICS	PARENTAL ROLE
Developing hearty appetites	Set regular meal and snack times

School-age

CHARACTERISTICS	PARENTAL ROLE
Becoming susceptible to peer pressure	Prepare healthy, nourishing meals
Being influenced by television advertising	Help children understand television advertising for high-sugar, high-fat, low-nutrient foods

Adolescence

CHILDREN'S DEVELOPMENT	PARENTAL ROLE
Becoming concerned about appearance	Provide nutritious food at home
Being influenced by TV advertising	Set a good example, especially for fast foods
Becoming very susceptible to peer pressure. May be experimenting with fad diets	Provide guidance; become informed about and be aware of the problem
Growing rapidly	

Source: The Yale Guide To Children's Nutrition, 1997

DISH IT OUT, AND LET THEM TAKE IT

Many experts say you shouldn't force your kid to eat new foods or even make them finish what's on their plate, but that's much, much easier said than done. The parent's only job is to put nutritious food on the table, and it's up to the kid to eat it or not to eat it, says Ellyn Satter, author of *How To Get Your Kid To Eat...But Not Too Much.*

That's not how many of our moms functioned. One friend recalls being told to clean her plate because there were "starving children in China." So she sat there painstakingly chewing a vegetable that tasted so foul, her stomach churned. With a mouth full of food, she barked back: "Oh yeah? Send them my Brussels sprouts."

Many parents, Satter writes, cross the line when they try to control the amount their children eat and when they don't prepare healthful meals. According to Satter, force-feeding occurs when you do the following:

- ◆ You try to get a child to eat more or less than she wants.

- ◆ You try to get your child to finish a vegetable he doesn't like.

- ◆ You short-order cook for your child because if you don't she will starve.

- ◆ You bribe your preteen with a cookie for eating certain foods.

Force-feeding is even less effective when your kids get older. You don't have as much control once they start going to school and spending their own money on snacks. Preteens are more fad-oriented and much more interested in becoming separate from their parents and emulating other adolescents. They are much more likely to stress their own independence in what they want to eat, so it's especially important to put them on a healthful track as early as possible.

ALL IN THE FAMILY

 Your child's ability to like some foods but not others may depend on her genetic makeup. Also, sometimes illnesses or allergies interfere with the ability to taste or smell certain foods. But mostly, children learn to eat foods that they are repeatedly exposed to. If you and your spouse enjoy mealtime, so will your children. But if you force them to eat, they'll develop negative associations with food and lose their ability to judge whether they are hungry.

SHORT-ORDER COOKING

If your kid won't eat anything, won't he starve? Not if you serve a variety of foods every night and set an example for good, nutritious eating. The worst thing to do, experts say, is to become your child's short-order cook. This reinforces his impression that he doesn't need to try anything new and gives you another meal to cook.

But some moms disagree with this theory. One mom said she thought of her family as guests. "I thought cooking what they like was being a good hostess," she told me. But she added, "back then I made my own baby food too…I wasn't working." If she had a job, she explains, she couldn't have provided so many food options.

My opinion on the short-order cook dilemma is to give your children the choice of eating what you are serving for the whole family most of the time. But once a week, make a meal just for them, where they can pick what they want. If they choose fried chicken with french fries, remember that you're eating it only once in a while. You don't want to go the opposite direction and prohibit everything that's unhealthy, because then your kids will want it more and will buy it secretly.

ALL IN THE FAMILY

 According to *American Academy of Pediatrics: Feeding Kids Right Isn't Always Easy*, parents and caregivers have five important feeding jobs:

- ◆ Offer a variety of healthful and tasty foods. Be adventurous.
- ◆ Serve meals and snacks on a regular schedule.
- ◆ Make mealtime pleasant.
- ◆ Teach good manners at the table.
- ◆ Set a good example.

YOU THINK YOUR KID IS FINICKY?

You are at a restaurant, and your kid lets out a shriek. The peas in his plate accidentally rolled into the rice. He refuses to eat his dinner. Or you give your child cucumbers, the only vegetable she likes, and she says: "Yuck, these are gross!" Every mother has a finicky story to tell about her kid. They may sound funny to others, but they're not funny to the mom trying to survive her child's eating habits.

Kids invent weird rules about what goes with what foods. For example, it's OK to have peas with steak, but not with chicken. French toast doesn't go with juice, just water. Sometimes, this finickiness is due to a medical problem. Take your child to the pediatrician to rule out that possibility. But most times, kids are just fussy by nature.

Experts say it's normal for children to go through finicky stages. This behavior is so common that someone took the time to come up with categories of finicky eaters. The American Academy of Pediatrics (AAP) breaks down the world of finicky eaters into six types and offers suggestions on how to deal with them. Your child may fit into one of these categories (or, if you're lucky, all of them).

Food Jags

Some kids want the same food for every single meal. According to the AAP, if what your child wants is wholesome, it's OK to let her eat it. Tell her other foods are available for her to eat, urge her to try just one bite of another food, and then let her decide. If she asks for fish sticks or other high-fat foods every day, let her eat them but serve different, healthy side dishes.

A research study showed that most children won't accept a new food until they've been exposed to it a dozen times. The first four meals, the kid looks at the food on the plate and pays no attention to it. Most parents give up offering new foods after one or two tries. You should, however, continue serving a variety of foods at dinner because without pressure (and a parent to fight with), your kids will eventually try other dishes.

Food Strikes

Some kids refuse to eat what you give them and then demand a special dinner. You dash to the kitchen to comply with these dictators' orders. You've become a short-order cook. It's not fun, but is it good for your child? Warning: If you cater to your child's demands, he may become even more picky because he realizes that wanting something entirely different is OK and watching Mom run around to accommodate him is fun.

No one wants you to starve your child, but the most you're risking is having your child miss an occasional meal. Tell him, "I'm sorry, this is what's being served tonight," and then offer him some of the items in the meal that may appeal to him. Remember, your only job is to serve a nutritious meal. Your child has to make his own decisions about what he'll eat. Eventually, he'll stop expecting everyone to cater to his needs.

The TV Habit

Some kids won't eat because they are too absorbed watching TV. Families should not watch TV or read the paper at dinnertime because it's one of the only times everyone gathers to catch up on the day. This hour is sacred, and it may be the glue that holds your family together. But if your kid is devastated by you turning off the TV, suggest that on a particular night, after dinner, the entire family sit together and watch something. If the show your kid likes is on during dinner, you could always tape it and watch it later.

The Complainer

Most parents go bonkers when their children not only refuse to eat, but also whine and complain. "No fair, why can't I eat something I like." "I don't want that food, it's gross." If your child is a complainer, tell her that she can't spoil everyone else's dinner and send her to her room until the meal is finished.

The Great American White Food Diet

Some kids are anti-color when it comes to food. They love to eat bread, potatoes, macaroni, and milk. How do you add some color to their life? Offer them rich-colored vegetables. Caving in to their needs by giving finicky eaters more attention reinforces a child's demands to limit foods.

Fear of New Foods

If your child is especially resistant to new foods, continue serving them. The child may take a while to try them, but he'll come around. When you put too much pressure on kids to try something new, they'll react by refusing to eat. The AAP recommends that you serve a food your children enjoy along with food they have refused to eat in the past. Try serving a food again if it was refused before. Remember: Sometimes kids have to see a food several times before they'll try it.

MOM ALWAYS SAID

Mom always said that kids will eat junk all day if given the option. A 1920's researcher, however, found that kids selected a good combination of the right foods when left on their own. But the researcher's spread was filled with healthful foods, not the candy, cookies, and other junk our kids would probably prefer to eat. So mom may have been right all along.

ARE PICKY EATERS JUST STUFFED?

When deciding whether your child is picky, consider other factors. Maybe your child isn't hungry because he's recently had a filling snack, maybe you've just dumped too much food on his plate for lunch, or maybe he just doesn't have to eat as much because he didn't get much exercise that afternoon. Parents often overestimate how much food a child from 5 to 12 requires. At this age, kids don't need adult-sized portions. Parents who don't realize this fact may be heaping too much food on their kids' plates and then criticizing them for not finishing it. Talk about adding insult to injury.

As the middle years move on, children's total energy requirements increase and they begin to need more food. Between ages 7 to 10, both boys and girls consume about 1,600 to 2,400 calories a day. Most girls have a higher growth rate between 10 to 12 and will take in about 200 more calories. Boys go through their growth spurt about two years later and then take in 500 additional calories a day. Your child will lose much of her finickiness when she begins her growth spurt. But until then, her tastes will remain unpredictable.

Don't worry if your child doesn't get all her nutrients in one day. What matters is that she eat lots of different things over the course of a couple of days. If you aren't sure she is getting it all, keep a diary of everything your child eats for a week. If your kid is energetic and productive after a week, she is getting all the energy she needs, regardless of whether she appears finicky to you. If your child appears lethargic or depressed, see your pediatrician to rule out any medical problems.

GIVE FASTIDIOUS EATERS OPTIONS

You don't have to race to the kitchen to make a special meal for your child when she refuses to eat what's on the table, but you shouldn't choose to make meals without any regard to her preferences. If your child's finickiness revolves around the colors of the foods, for example, you can honor that and try to serve some alternatives:

- If green vegetables repulse your kids, try deep-yellow or orange vegetables or hide vegetables in food. You can throw peas, carrots, and other veggies in soups and meat pies, or add shredded lettuce to sandwiches.

- If you've got anti-fruit kids, then give them a milkshake made with chopped fresh fruit, ice, and nonfat frozen yogurt.

- If your kids don't like mushy vegetables, give them crunchy veggies with a dip.

- If your kids don't want milk, give them low-fat chocolate milk, cheese, or yogurt.

- If they don't want to eat beef and pork, try giving them chicken, ground turkey, or fish.

◆ If they refuse bread and cereal, try giving them warm cereal and add raisins or fruit on top. If this combination doesn't peak their interest, give them more pasta and rice. These items have the same nutrients as bread and cereal and are from the same food group.

DON'T USE DESSERTS AS THREATS OR REWARDS

How many times have you heard (or said) something like the following?

◆ "If you don't eat your chicken, you can't have dessert."

◆ "If you behave, I'll get you an ice cream cone."

◆ "Eat everything on your plate, and then you can get cookies."

These threats and rewards flow out of our mouths as easily as our names. We say them because our mothers said them, because we hear other moms say them, because we can't imagine how else to get our kids to eat right. Does it work?

Most of us think it works, at least in the short term. Your kid complains, but wolfs down his vegetables anticipating his cake. But the experts think we are doing it all wrong. They say that using desserts or treats for eating more nutritious foods is not the way to go. If kids are constantly getting cake as a reward for eating their spinach, they will see the cake as the more important and better food than the vegetable.

Parents, experts tell us, should try to ingrain in their children a love for all foods. This way, they don't have to resort to force-feeding. How do you shift gears from using desserts as leverage to a more sensible approach? The easy answer is to make dessert as healthful as everything else and to get rid of the high-fat cookies and candies in your cupboard. Offer strawberries or other fruits for dessert and top them off with yogurt. Some parents serve dessert with the meal so that all parts of the meal are equal, instead of dessert being the best. To some parents' surprise, kids eat the dessert first, realize they are still hungry, and delve into the rest of the meal.

TURN PERSNICKETY KIDS INTO COOKS

One way you can get your preteen or teen to become less finicky is to get him to buy the food and/or cook it himself. Kids are curious by nature, and they like to taste what they create. If they become part of the decision-making process, they'll be more apt to try different foods, as long they are not being pressured or forced to eat anything. Kids also like to feel useful, and being in the kitchen is their chance to look and act like an adult. For parents, this time is ideal for teaching your children about nutrition.

If you have the time, and your kids have the energy, take them to the store with you (see Chapters 3 and 4). You can teach them how to read labels and compare products. While strolling down the aisle, explain the importance of making lower fat choices when possible, such as choosing chicken over red meat.

When your children help you cook, make sure that whatever task you give them is age-appropriate. Your 8-year old may be too young to take a baked dish from the oven, but she can practice safety precautions by putting on the mitts and opening up the oven door. Kids can help cut up vegetables, measure and mix ingredients, and put meals together. Who knows? Maybe they'll learn to cook so well that in a couple of years you'll come home and they'll have dinner ready on the table! (A mom can fantasize, can't she?)

MOM KNOWS BEST

When you teach your kids to cook, start out by encouraging them to make simple foods involving one or two steps, such as popcorn, french toast, and garlic bread. Then move on to baking, boiling, and steaming. And then, the moment all moms have been waiting for: Let your kids read recipes and make a meal. Regardless of how the food comes out, always praise them for trying and cheer them on to try again.

GET EVERYONE ON BOARD

A kid who is finicky to start with will have a harder time trying new foods if her parents aren't eating healthy, either. You or your partner, however, may find it difficult to stop eating high-fat foods. If you are trying to get your kid to stop eating high-fat desserts, but your husband is serving himself a large plate of cake with ice cream on top, you'll have a tough time answering, "If Daddy has some, why can't I?"

Your husband may never ask the waitress to substitute T-bone with tofu, but he could be more open than you think about changing his lifestyle to a healthier one. You can start campaigning by doing the following:

- Explain to your partner the importance of eating healthy. Tell him how eating high-fat, high-cholesterol diets can bring on heart disease and certain cancers.

- Explain that switching to a low-fat diet won't be as hard as everyone thinks; the meals won't be that different (look at Chapter 5 for sample substitutions).

- Suggest that the family team up and switch to healthier foods for one month to see how it works out.

If your partner's resistance turns to resentment for pushing this issue too far, let it go. There is more to good health than food. Make sure your child gets exercise, plenty of sleep, and lots of good family time. Having a stable family is more important to your child's health than eating whole-wheat bread. Your child's finicky problems may persist, or they just may go away as you stop pressuring your spouse and child about food.

THE LEAST YOU NEED TO KNOW

- Forcing kids to eat can lead to food disorders.

- Give fussy kids a choice of what foods they want to eat.

- Don't use dessert as a reward; doing so lowers the value of healthful entrees.

- Try asking your finicky kid to help you cook. She may like to eat foods she's cooked herself.

- Fussy kids eat better when their parents eat a healthy diet.

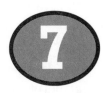

7

Fast, Faster, Fastest Food

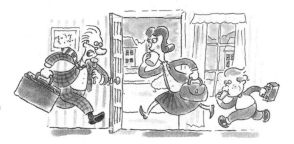

Eating out has become commonplace. Too tired to cook after schlepping your kids to dance class and karate? Take your kids out to eat. Nothing good to munch on? Go take the kids to get a milkshake. Don't feel like doing dishes after dinner? Go make a mess elsewhere. Sounds good to me.

But going out to eat can wreak havoc on your kids' arteries unless you select the foods carefully. This chapter tells you what types of healthful snacks-on-the-run your kids should eat and what to order at fast-food chains and restaurants so kids can get a treat filled with vitamins, minerals, nutrients, and flavor.

SNACKS: DON'T SPOIL YOUR APPETITE

"Don't eat those cookies," your parents probably told you, "they'll spoil your appetite." You grew up hearing that and maybe you now say the same thing to your kids. Why should they eat between meals? You don't!

The answer is simple: Most kids ages 8 to 14 need more calories than you do, and they can't get them from three meals. Snacks are an important part of your children's diets. Most children get nearly 25 percent of their nutritional requirements through snacks. Most teenagers skip breakfast, so snacks become even more important for them.

You still have some control over snacks with your school-age children, but many preteens and teens snack away from home and away from your watchful eye. Many teens rush into McDonald's for a Big Mac to munch on or grab some chips and dip for a quick bite. Such snack foods are high in calories, salt, sugar, and fat. All you can do is to keep reinforcing the importance of eating healthy, nutritious meals and hope this message will stick with your kids in the future.

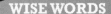

WISE WORDS

A nutritious snack contains protein, vitamins, and minerals, and is low in fat, sugar, and salt. Such snacks are also not excessively high in calories.

Buy Healthy Snacks

Tread the cookie aisle with caution. You'll be assaulted by cookies, cakes, and crackers whose boxes claim one spectacular thing or another—low-fat, nonfat, low-sodium. Read the label (see Chapter 3) to make sure you are selecting the best item for your children. Remember that reduced-fat varieties of high-fat snacks are not such great deals.

You can eliminate some snack items right off the bat: doughnuts, fried pastries, high-fat cookies, and pies. Palm kernel oil and coconut oil, two highly saturated vegetable fats, are often used to make crackers, chips, cookies, cake mixes, and granola bars.

Candies made with hydrogenated fats and chocolate are also high in fat. An eight-ounce bag of regular potato chips has about six tablespoons of oil and up to 80 grams of fat, about twice the amount of fat calories your child is supposed to have a day. The following are some healthier snacking alternatives.

Healthy Snacking	
INSTEAD OF	*HAVE SOME*
Ice cream	Nonfat frozen yogurt, popsicles, sorbets, fruit bars, frozen grapes
High-fat cakes	Angel-food cake topped with fruit
Buttered popcorn	Air-popped popcorn sprinkled with butter-flavored spray
Potato chips	Pretzels, low-fat chips
Chocolate cookies	Graham crackers, fig bars, vanilla wafers
Doughnuts, pastries	Bagels, English muffins

Other nutritious snacks include the following:

◆ Low-fat granola bars, oatmeal cookies

◆ Pudding made with skim milk

◆ Rice cakes, whole-grain crackers

◆ Dried fruits, fresh juices

◆ Raw vegetables with dip

◆ Peanuts (Two tablespoons of peanut butter have 14 grams of fat—with 2.5 g coming from saturated fats. The good news is that nearly 80% of fat is unsaturated.)

Make Quick, Easy, Nutritious Snacks

I know you have virtually no time to make dinner, so a suggestion that you also make nutritious snacks may sound off the wall. But if you want to take some time out on a weekend, take your child shopping and make some easy snacks together. This way, your child can learn about ingredients, cooking, and trying new foods.

Here are some easy recipes:

◆ Fill celery sticks with peanut butter.

◆ Cut up small pieces of cantaloupes, grapes, and strawberries and put them in a large ice cream cone.

◆ Serve cut-up fruits and vegetables with toothpicks.

◆ Slice some yams or potatoes into french-fry shapes, spread them on a lightly oiled cookie sheet and bake. Add whatever spices you like.

◆ Spray a tortilla with a little olive-oil mist, add some spices and low-fat cheese, then wrap it up and bake it.

Regulate Snack Time

Kids need snacks; otherwise, they just can't last from one meal to the next. But, like mom said, you don't want them to spoil their appetite. So what do you do? Plan their snacks just as you would map out their meals. If you are home, let your child eat a snack far enough in advance so she'll be hungry again by dinner. If you pick her up after-school and you know you won't be serving dinner for another hour, give her a piece of fruit to tide her over.

Also, consider the calories of the foods your child is snacking on. Higher calories will fill her up more and may affect her desire to eat at dinner time. If dinner is a half an hour away, better give her carrots to munch on (carrots are low-calorie) rather than a bagel.

SCHOOL LUNCHES: STILL LOUSY AFTER ALL THESE YEARS?

Remember the school lunches you ate when you were a kid? Meatloaf floating in muddy gravy, lumpy mashed potatoes, corn drowning in butter? The only foods that looked edible were the fried chicken, french fries, hot dogs, and potato chips. Everyone grabbed cake and brownies, instead of the bruised apple squatting next to a lonely orange. Have school lunches changed?

Over the past decade, school lunches have been heavily criticized for being loaded with fats, saturated fats, and sodium. But thanks to a law passed in 1995, which requires federally subsidized school lunches to meet the current dietary guidelines, today's lunch menu must now contain no more than 30 percent of total calories from fat and no more than 10 percent from saturated fats. That's an improvement, for sure, but a la carte menus are still high in fat.

The USDA's Team Nutrition, a group which teaches children, schools, and the public how to make healthful food choices, suggests that parents keep tabs on what kids eat at school:

◆ Eat breakfast or lunch at school with your kids to see what their meals are like. If you don't like it, do something. Talk to other parents, the PTA, and the school board to push for healthier meals.

◆ Talk to the principal about the importance of good nutrition and physical activity. Ask him or her to back your request for a change in meal plans.

◆ Get a weekly menu of school meals so you know what your kid is eating at lunch. Ask the school for a nutritional breakdown of the foods served to make sure the menu meets the official Dietary Guidelines for Americans (see Chapter 1). Talk to your kids about which foods are better for them.

◆ Ask your kids what they are learning at school about good nutrition, and then give them a chance to put that information into good use at home.

If your kid insists on eating a high-fat school lunch one day, plan to have a lighter, lower-fat dinner and give her healthier snacks, such as pretzels, fruits, or low-fat yogurt. Remind her to always order skim or one percent milk and take fruit instead of dessert. (But don't have unrealistic expectations that she'll dutifully obey you.)

MOM KNOWS BEST

If you are horrified at the quality of your school's lunches, bring it up at the next PTA meeting and keep voicing your concerns until the administration agrees to splatter more nutritious foods on your child's plate.

Brown-Bagging It

If your child is going to take his lunch, make his meal not only balanced and nutritious, but also exciting. Your kids, like many kids, could probably subsist on peanut butter and jelly sandwiches for a long time. But eventually they'll get sick of the same old lunch and will either throw it out or trade it for something with more pizzazz. School lunches for school-age kids should include the following:

♦ At least two servings from the grain group

♦ One fruit or vegetable

♦ One serving from the meat or dairy groups (try to stay away from high-fat processed meats, included in many packaged lunches)

♦ Some kind of snack or dessert (optional)

How you want to combine these food groups is up to you. Try giving your children different types of sandwiches to limit the use of eggs and peanut butter to three or four times a week. To keep fat intake down, use low-fat cheeses, reduced-calorie mayonnaise or salad dressing, and sandwich spreads such as mustard and chili sauce that are low in fat.

Giant Supermarket publishes a guide to packing nutritious lunches. Here are some of its suggestions to jazz up sandwiches:

♦ Top cheese sandwiches with sliced cucumber, onion, and alfalfa sprouts

♦ Add raisins, grated carrot, sliced apples, or chopped dates to peanut butter sandwiches

♦ Mix chopped, hard-boiled eggs or mashed tofu with mustard and low-fat mayo

◆ Mix tuna fish (packed in water) with low-fat mayo and plain non-fat yogurt and add celery, green pepper, apples, or raisins

◆ Use processed lunch meats with no more than one gram of fat per ounce or that are labeled 95 to 99 percent fat-free.

Many of us dreaded eating lunch at school. After all, what was there to look forward to? The same old peanut butter and jelly sandwich? Colorless foods served at the cafeteria by dour lunch personnel? But you can make lunch fun for your kid by mixing and matching foods. No guarantee he'll eat it, but at least you are fulfilling your job—to provide healthful meals.

Sandwichless in the School Cafeteria

Most of us make school lunches when we are least creative: either at night before going to sleep or when we are in a complete rush, early in the morning. So what do we make? Sandwiches. The same sandwiches, day in and day out, until our kids gripe: "Not again, I want something else."

What else is there to give them? How about sandwichless lunches? Giant Supermarket came up with some fun, delicious alternatives to the sandwich:

◆ A hard-boiled egg left in the shell

◆ Barbecued chicken drumsticks or slices of turkey on top of a tossed salad

◆ Cubes of cheese and meat with celery, grapes, or crunchy apples in a container

◆ Leftover chili, soup, or stew in a thermos—either hot or cold

◆ A lettuce "sandwich:" roll your kid's favorite filling in a large lettuce leaf or wrap meat slices around pickles, cucumber, or zucchini and secure with toothpick

◆ A wedge of leftover pizza

◆ Green or red peppers or cored apples stuffed with cottage cheese and mixed with raisins or chopped vegetables

◆ Yogurt, either plain or with cut-up fruit and dry cereal sprinkled on top

Who could imagine such lunch varieties without slapping two pieces of bread at each end? Being a little creative can take you a long way, especially with feeding school-age children and teens. And once you get into the swing of thinking about alternative foods, you'll never go back to the boring days of throwing plain old peanut butter and jelly in the lunch bag.

Anything for Dessert?

It's easy to go to the food warehouse and buy a box of 40 bags of potato chips, cartons of cookies, and cupcakes, especially with your child begging for them. But these items are nutritional zeros. Choose snacks like fruits (both fresh and dried), fruit-filled shredded wheat cereals, pretzels, and low-fat yogurt.

As for desserts? Avoid prepackaged puddings, cakes, and other convenient snacks because these are high in saturated fats, sugar, and additives. Instead, give your children graham crackers, oatmeal-raisin cookies, and other low-fat cookies.

ALL IN THE FAMILY

 If you don't want to drive yourself crazy, avoid making lunches at the last minute. Mornings are hectic: Kids refuse to get out of bed, and when they do, they're grumpy, they can't decide what to wear, and don't want anything you offer for breakfast. Meanwhile, you're late for work.

Prepare lunches the night before and refrigerate them. To keep the food safe, use insulated lunch boxes (which hold the cold better than bags). Also use small plastic tubs from yogurt, margarine, and other foods to carry salads and fruits. To prevent cut fruits from turning brown, dip them in lemon, orange, or grapefruit juice before packing them up. If you're packing dairy or mayonnaise-based foods, it's safer to include a dry-ice packet in the lunch box to keep the food from spoiling.

FAST FOODS: PLEASE PASS THE GREASE

Everything you do is on the run. You snack on the run, shop on the run, talk to friends on the run. And when you are worn out from running, you come home to starving children and then pile back into the car to make a run for another fast-food dinner. The National Restaurant Association says that Americans dole out about $800 million each day on foods eaten away from home. Eating out used to be reserved for special occasions; now the special occasion is eating at home.

The fact is that as long as there are busy people, fast-food chains will thrive. Most moms look at the food options and groan. Fast-food restaurants cater to what they think are children's palates, using high-fat foods, excess sugar, and lots of salt.

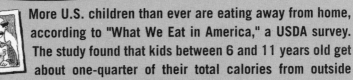

ALL IN THE FAMILY

More U.S. children than ever are eating away from home, according to "What We Eat in America," a USDA survey. The study found that kids between 6 and 11 years old get about one-quarter of their total calories from outside food. Kids between 12 and 19 get about one-third of their daily calories from restaurants and fast-food outlets. Kids' favorite fast-food fare includes pizza, tacos, and burritos.

Greasy Foods Your Kids Love to Eat

Look over this list of how many calories and fat calories your children's favorite foods contain:

Hope S. Warshaw, author of *The Restaurant Companion: A Guide to Healthier Eating Out* (Surrey Books, Inc., 1995), looks into just how many calories and fat calories your children's favorite foods contain:

◆ A Big Mac, 510 calories, 46% fat.

◆ McDonald's French Fries (large), 450 calories, 44% fat

◆ Hardee's Hot Dog, 450 calories, 40% fat.

- Wendy's Chocolate Chip Cookie, 270 calories, 37% fat.

- One slice of Domino's cheese pizza, 280 calories, 39% fat.

- McDonald's Egg McMuffin, 290 calories, 40% fat.

- Denny's Steak & Eggs, 800 calories, 57% fat.

- Dunkin' Donuts Jelly-filled doughnut, 220 calories, 37% fat.

- Carl's Junior breakfast burrito, 430 calories, 54% fat.

Going out to eat at your kid's hangout sounds like a grease-feast! Yuck! But most of these restaurants have awakened to Americans' health concerns and are offering low-fat options. Now, if we could only get our kid to stare at someone else's Big Mac while happily eating their grilled chicken alternatives.

ALL IN THE FAMILY

Of nearly 66 million Americans who eat out at least one meal a day, 33 percent choose fast-food restaurants. The New England Journal of Medicine said that nearly 40 percent to 55 percent of the typical fast-food meal is made out of fat. Even nutritious foods, such as baked potatoes, are turned to fat with added toppings such as sour cream and bacon bits. Fast-food chains spend nearly one billion a year on television advertising, and our kids eat every bite.

Fast-Food Chains Offer Low-Fat Options

Not all fast-food chains are nutritional death traps. Many fast-food chains now offer foods with lower calories, lower fat content, and more fiber. In her book, Warshaw suggests that you inch away from the high-fat foods into leaner alternatives a little bit at a time. A McLean Deluxe at McDonald's, for instance, has 342 calories, 32 percent fat—better for you than a Big Mac.

You'd be better off with a Burger King's Broiler Chicken Sandwich, at 540 calories, 48 percent fat, than with a fried chicken sandwich. You could order your child an Arby's Junior Roast Beef (233 calories, 42 percent fat), rather than splurging with a Giant Roast Beef, which rings in at 544 calories, 43 percent fat. And you can do even better! A chicken breast sandwich at Boston Market has only 422 calories, 9 percent fat. Wendy's Grilled Chicken is 290 calories, 22 percent fat.

MOM KNOWS BEST

Most fast-food chains now offer salad bars, roasted chicken, baked potatoes, low-cal dressings, and other lower-fat items. Foods called Jumbo, Double Whopper, or Super-Size usually have more mayonnaise, dressings, pickles, and fatty meats than regular-size items. If you order fish or chicken, make sure they are roasted, baked, or broiled rather than buttered and fried. If your kid is a nuggets addict, cut back on calories by avoiding high-fat—usually cream-based—sauces (or using the sauces sparingly). The focus should be on lower fat, not necessarily lower calories, unless your child is obese.

DON'T KNOCK NUTRITION IN RESTAURANTS

If you can't stand the thought of going to a fast-food restaurant but you still don't want to cook at home, go to a "family-style" restaurant, a cut above fast-food joints, where your dinners are served at the table by people who say hello to you. In these restaurants, you and your kids can easily ask for substitutions to make your meals healthier. Look for low-fat dishes, which include anything steamed, broiled, baked, grilled, poached, or roasted. If you don't know how a dish is made, ask. If the menu doesn't have a section of light entrees, don't give up. Ask if your meal can be prepared with leaner cuts of meat or request that sauces or dressings come on the side.

If you're nervous about going to a restaurant with your family and getting stuck with high-fat meals, look over the menu before you go, or call the restaurant directly. In the pamphlet "Tips For Eating Out," the National Heart Association suggests that you ask the following questions:

◆ Will the restaurant honor special food preparation requests?

◆ Can food be prepared without salt and MSG?

◆ Can dressings and sauces be served on the side?

◆ Can margarine rather than butter be served with the meal?

◆ Does the restaurant serve skim or one percent milks rather than whole milk?

◆ Can dishes be prepared with vegetable oil (canola, olive, corn, soy, sunflower, safflower) or margarine made with vegetable oil?

◆ Will the chef trim visible fat from meat and remove the skin from poultry before cooking?

◆ Will the chef broil, bake, steam, or poach rather than fry foods?

◆ Can the chef leave all butter, gravy, or sauces off entrees and side dishes?

◆ Does the menu include fruit, ices, sherbet, or nonfat frozen yogurt for dessert?

If you ask me, that's a lot of questions to ask for just a quick little meal! I mean, if you're going to go through the hassle of doing all this research ahead of time, why not devote that to meal preparation at home?

Unless your child has food sensitivities or severe weight problems, you can limit yourself to four basic questions:

◆ What types of fats are used to prepare meals? (Stick to foods made with predominantly unsaturated fats that come from corn oil, safflower oil, sesame oil, peanut oil, olive oil, canola oil.)

◆ What cooking methods are used? Best methods for meat, fish, and poultry are baking, broiling, grilling, poaching, roasting, and boiling. Vegetables should be microwaved, steamed, or stir-fried.

◆ What is the sauce made of? The best sauces are those reduced from vegetable or chicken broth, as opposed to those made from cream or fat.

◆ Which cuts of meat are used? Go for lean cuts that have less fat. (When you order ground beef, ask for extra-lean hamburger or ground round. The light meat on poultry also has less fat.)

DON'T RESORT TO FAT FOODS AT RESORTS

You are finally going away for a week to one of those fabulous resorts where your kids can swim, bike, hike, and enjoy every meal on their kids' menu, consisting basically of four items: chicken nuggets, hot dogs, hamburgers, and pasta. The pasta is OK, but the rest of the items don't exactly fit into your healthful eating schedule. What do you do, throw nutrition out the window? Not necessarily. Debbie Daley, director of Nutrition Services at the Spa Doral, suggests that the parents get appetizers for themselves and then share healthful entrees with their children.

She also suggests that parents keep in mind what their kids eat throughout the day. If your kid wants a hamburger with fries for lunch, tell him that if he has that now he can't have another burger for dinner. Instead, offer him a turkey sandwich or another lower-fat option. The goal is to balance foods, not withhold all grease.

Daley also recommends that if possible, you go to a nearby supermarket and buy fresh fruits, carrots, and other snacks you can keep handy for nibbling during the day instead of buying potato chips, nachos, ice cream, and other poolside options that add fat and calories to your day.

DEVELOP SALAD SAVVY

You may feel proud of your children if they choose salads as their meals. After all, salads are an excellent source of fiber and vitamins A and C. But lurking amid the beans, lettuce, tomatoes, and other nutritious food are high-fat culprits: tuna salad, egg salad, bacon bits, and other foods that raise red flags.

So when your children make a beeline to the buffet, make sure they load their plate with fresh veggies, whole grains, and low-fat dressings. Teach them to pile on lettuces, especially spinach and romaine, all fresh vegetables, a small scoop of low-fat cottage cheese (full of calcium and protein), and other low-sodium, low-fat foods.

In addition, make sure they don't ruin the nutritious effect of these foods by pouring on ladles of prepared dressings, bacon bits, and croutons—the bad guys hiding in the buffet. The following is a partial list of high-calorie and high-sodium products at a typical

American salad bar, prepared by the U.S. Department of Agriculture, Human Nutrition Information Service.

Calories and Sodium at the American Salad Bar		
FOOD	CALORIES (PER 100 GRAMS OR 3 1/2 OUNCES)	SODIUM (MILLIGRAMS PER 100 GRAMS)
Bacon bits	530	3,065
Black olives	150	230
Broccoli	25	12
Carrots	40	33
Cheese, shredded	380	1,125
Croutons	390	735
Cucumber	10	6
Olives, green	95	680
Pickles	65	1,970
Potato salad	145	480
Spinach	22	50
Tomato	20	4

Source: Excerpts of the U.S. Department of Agriculture, Human Nutrition Information Service.

Salad dressings offered at salad bars (usually creamy blue cheese, thousand island, creamy ranch, or Italian) tend to be high in fat, although we are beginning to see more low-fat or fat-free alternatives. Urge your child to use regular dressings sparingly. The best option is to just sprinkle a dab of oil and vinegar in the salad.

ETHNIC FOODS FIT FOR YOUR KIDS

At some point, you may feel the need to put your foot down and say, "No, we are not going to McDonald's again this week." First, the choice of nutritious foods is limited at fast-food places. Second, you may be tired of having nothing good to eat. Third, you've seen enough of Americana all day—you may be ready for something exotic, exciting, and different.

Ethnic foods may be the option you are looking for. Most kids have lots of exposure to Chinese, Mexican, or Italian foods, and these foods, give or take a few sauces, can be healthy. Teaching your kids to taste foods from around the world is an important part of getting your kids to try new foods. The following tips will help you figure out which foods will benefit your children, how you can turn unhealthy meals into nutritious ones, and which dishes your child is likely to enjoy the most.

Stir-Fry Chinese Stirs the Palate

Chinese food is so different and exciting that even kids who don't like their foods to touch may suspend their finickiness somewhat to enjoy this cuisine. Because many dishes contain meat, chicken, lots of veggies, and rice, this cuisine is nutritious as well. Most foods are quickly cooked on a wok with unsaturated oils, which means many of the nutrients are retained.

But the sauces and too much oil can kill a good thing. Avoid ordering deep-fried dishes, those that have heavy sauces (lobster, sweet and sour, hoisin), and those prepared with monosodium glutamate (MSG). The following list gives you some more info on what to order and what to avoid.

Ordering Chinese Foods	
RESIST THESE:	*ORDER THESE:*
Sweet and sour pork	Stir-fried or steamed chicken or fish
Egg rolls	Stir-fried or steamed meat

continues

Ordering Chinese Foods (continued)	
RESIST THESE:	*ORDER THESE:*
Egg foo yung	Stir-fried or steamed tofu and vegetables
Deep-fried chicken	Vegetable platters with sauces, mushrooms, bamboo shoots, snow peas, and other vegetables
Fried rice	Steamed white rice
Spare ribs	Fortune cookies
Fried dumplings	Steamed dumplings
Seafood with lobster sauce	Cold noodles with sesame sauce

Spice Up Your Kid's Life with Mexican Foods

Mexican restaurants are popular with kids who like the festive decor, the exotic music, the messy food—the sheer loudness! As soon as you sit down to order, they start fighting over the chips. Now, salsa they can eat to their heart's delight. But chips...not really. You can either remove the chips from the table (since kids fill up on these and you get stuck with a high bill and full plates), or, more reasonably, you can divide the chips up among the kids and tell the waiter "no thank you," when he asks if you want a refill.

Mexican cuisine can fit into any reduced-fat eating plan, if you order properly. Mexican food can be perfectly nutritious because so many dishes, particularly those made with rice, vegetables, tortillas, and legumes (remember those guys?), are high in fiber and complex carbohydrates. Many other foods, however, are bloated with fat and sodium.

As in all other restaurants, ask what's in the food, and don't be afraid to ask for substitutions. Choose soft corn tortillas instead of fried tortilla chips. Stick with cheeseless entrees and low-fat meats.

Ordering Mexican Foods

RESIST THESE:	*ORDER THESE:*
Tacos or burritos made with refried beans, beef, or cheese	Fajitas made with marinated lean beef or chicken with vegetables
Nachos	Vegetable quesadillas
Refried beans	Mexican rice
Sour cream, guacamole	Use salsa or salsa verde
Fried tortillas	Soft taco shells
Beef and cheese enchiladas	Fish or chicken marinated in lime juice
Chimichangas	Gazpacho Corn tortillas with salsa Chicken tostada Cheeseless burritos

Italian Foods—That's Amore!

Ask your kids about their favorite foods, and many will say pizza and pasta. These foods are perfect for kids because they come with a variety of toppings, shapes, and sauces. Plain pizza provides many of the nutrients your kids need. Toss fresh veggies on the pizza, like green peppers, onions, and mushrooms, and you'll add vitamin C and fiber. The combination of cheese, crust, and tomato sauce delivers significant amounts of calcium, protein, riboflavin, thiamin, niacin, iron, and vitamin A. Let your kids enjoy plain pasta and pizza as long as possible because it won't be long before they savor the taste of other Italian foods that are not as healthful.

Ordering Italian Foods

RESIST THESE:	ORDER THESE:
Antipasto	Minestrone soup
Garlic bread	Plain warm bread or bread sticks with sprinkled cheese
Alfredo and pesto sauces	Marinara or plain tomato sauce
Cheese-filled lasagna, veal parmigiana, and cannelloni	Pizza with cheese and vegetable toppings
Meatballs	Boneless chicken
Cream pastries	Italian ice

THE LEAST YOU NEED TO KNOW

♦ Fruits, veggies, and crackers make nutritious snacks.

♦ Make school lunches exciting by offering sandwichless choices like salads, soups, stews, and mixed fruits.

♦ Order low-fat options at fast-food chains.

♦ Ask for healthful substitutes at restaurants.

♦ Stay away from bacon, croutons, and mayo-filled foods at salad bars.

♦ Chinese, Mexican, and Italian cuisines can be healthful if you stay away from foods that are fried or served in high-calorie sauces.

8

Jock Food

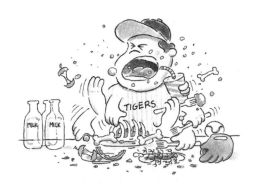

Your athletic child dreams of being a great baseball player, but unless he maintains a healthy diet, he probably won't hit too many home runs. Unfortunately, many of us get so caught up with our kids' athletic competition that we don't focus on their nutrition.

Who can worry about carbo grams when your son was just thrown on the bench by a coach who is an idiot? Can you think about dehydration when your daughter's wrists just slipped off the parallel bars at a varsity competition? Clearly, meals take a back seat during game season. But in order for children to succeed in sports, they must eat the right foods and drink plenty of fluids before, during, and after exercise.

Don't get too carried away. It's OK to charge to McDonald's once in a while with the rest of the gang to wolf down burgers or to take your daughter out for ice cream to celebrate a victory. Just keep an eye on your athlete's intake. Child athletes need to eat everything their more sedentary friends eat, especially low-fat, low-cholesterol foods and plenty of fruits and vegetables, plus extra calories to keep ahead of the race.

This chapter deals with what you can do to ensure that your young jocks eat the foods they need to play hard and that enough fluids are sloshing in their bellies when they are shooting hoops, swinging from parallel bars, or kicking the soccer ball into the goal.

WATCH JOCKS GROW

Most kids don't think that what they eat affects their athletic performance. Boys and girls are more concerned about how they look and who looks at them.

Boys check for bulging muscles and hope their bodies will get bigger so they can slam dunk a basketball and strut their stuff in front of their friends. Some are in such a hurry to grow that they take supplements and drugs to puff themselves up. But most boys don't realize that they ain't gonna hustle muscle until their bodies become sexually mature. Only time, and hormones, will build their body mass, weight, and strength, and eating nutritious foods will help them along the way.

Girls, on the other hand, usually want to trim down. Many girls resort to weight-reduction pills, vomiting, and other unhealthy techniques to keep their weight down, a dangerous approach that can often lead to eating disorders (see Chapter 11).

CALORIE COUNTING FOR ATHLETES

Most teen athletes need about 500 to 1,500 extra calories a day to give them the energy to practice and compete. That means that a teenager who normally needs 2,800 calories a day should devour up to 4,300 calories. Teens who walk, bike, or participate in other low- to moderate-intensity sports probably only need about 500 extra calories. Those who are involved in more intense activities need closer to 1,500 extra calories.

How many calories do teens expend on different sports? According to the *Yale Guide to Children's Nutrition* (1997, Yale University), a 110-pound adult basketball player burns 6.9 calories per minute and 414 calories an hour. Football jocks expend 6.6 calories per minute and 396 calories an hour. A tennis athlete burns 5.5 calories per minute and 330 calories an hour. The total calorie expenditure for gymnastics is 3.3 per minute and 196 an hour.

You won't have to beg your athlete to eat additional calories. She'll automatically eat more because she'll be hungrier after all her activities. Plus, practice often cuts into eating time, so she'll eat more snacks than most kids do throughout the day.

This schedule is less than ideal for working moms who want some control over their kids' diets. The best you can do is to feed your children healthful foods at home and hope that they will continue to choose a healthy eating style when they're away from home. You can't run into the middle of the soccer game with a bowl of fruit, but you can serve fruit for dessert at home.

EXTRA CARBOS FUEL YOUR JOCK'S ENGINE

Carbohydrates are an excellent fuel to rev up your jock's engine; this nutritious energy source should make up between 50 to 55 percent of your kid's total calories. To translate calories into grams, divide the number of calories (say 1,500) by 4 (because 1 gram of carbohydrates equals 4 calories). Thus the active basketball player needs to eat an extra 375 grams of carbohydrates to pack in extra fuel for energy.

Don't go bonkers thinking you've got to start reorganizing the family meals to accommodate the additional carbohydrates. Just throw open your cupboard and the carbohydrate grams will stare you in the face—pretzels, rice, muffins, spaghetti, and other complex carbo foods your athlete will eat in a snap.

The following are some examples of foods that are high in carbohydrates from each food group:

- Grain group: bagels, English muffins, oatmeal, pancakes, pretzels, flour tortillas, cereal, pasta, angel food cake, granola bars

- Fruit group: applesauce, cherries, cantaloupes, grape juice, prunes, raisins, watermelon

- Vegetable group: corn, carrots, white potatoes, sweet potatoes, peas

- Dairy group: low-fat frozen yogurt, skim milk, pudding

MORE PROTEINS DON'T PUSH JOCKS TO GO THE EXTRA MILE

If you are dishing out steak and eggs to your daughter before her big game, you need to rethink your efforts. True, athletic kids need more protein than their couch potato friends, but Americans already eat way more protein than they need—one and a half times the recommended daily allowance (RDA). The amount of protein your kids eat now is probably enough to help them build and maintain muscle tissue, including muscles that get banged out of shape while working out.

According to the American Dietetic Association (ADA), an athlete's protein needs are the following:

- Boys and girls ages 7 to 10 need 28 grams of protein.

- Boys 11 to 14 need 45 grams of protein.

- Girls 11 to 14 need 46 grams of protein.

Now check out the protein grams in the following foods:

- One cup of low-fat milk has 8 grams of protein.

- Three ounces of chicken, lean meat, or fish (a serving the size of a deck of cards) has 21 grams.

- Two tablespoons of peanut butter has 9 grams.

- Eight ounces of low-fat plain yogurt has 12 grams.

- Three and a half ounces of tuna canned in water has 28 grams.

- Half a cup of low-fat cottage cheese has 155 grams.

Ensuring that your athlete is getting enough proteins shouldn't be hard. American children get more protein than they need a day—what they don't get enough of is fruits, vegetables and grains. So if you want the kid to run the extra mile, give him carbos and skip McDonald's.

ALL IN THE FAMILY

Your 6 to 10 year old probably needs to eat about .5 grams of protein per pound of body weight each day. Growing teenage athletes need more protein, .6 to .9 grams per pound. A 13-year old gymnast who weighs 92 pounds, for instance, needs 43-60 grams of protein each day. You can supply the extra grams in an extra glass of milk or serving of meat.

Vegetarian Jocks

If your kid loves baseball, but hates barbecues, what's a mom to do? Back in Chapter 2, I discussed how animal proteins have all nine amino acids your kid needs. If your kid does not eat meat or dairy products, he may end up with serious deficiencies unless he closely watches his diet. His diet may lack:

◆ Vitamin B12, found in animal sources and in some fortified cereals

◆ Calcium, consumed in milk and other dairy products

◆ Iron, which is not absorbed as well from plant sources as it is from animal sources

But moms of vegetarian athletes shouldn't panic. Come up with some plant food combinations that string along all nine amino acids. Some examples:

◆ Rice and beans

◆ Tortillas and beans

◆ Whole-wheat bread and peanut butter

Just because your child isn't a meat eater it doesn't mean he can't be on the soccer team. For more details concerning feeding a vegetarian child see Chapter 9, "Jump on the Veggie Bandwagon."

TOO MUCH FAT RUINS THE FUN

Young athletes may be special when it comes to sports, but that doesn't mean they can handle fatty foods any better than slouchy, middle-aged adults. When it comes to grub, we are all bound by the same rules: Everyone over age two should stick to a diet made up of 30 percent fat (less than 10 percent of which should come from saturated fats) and under 300 grams of cholesterol.

But don't deprive your child of fat either. After all, fat is a concentrated form of energy, and kids need a lot of energy to play sports. Carbohydrates, though, do most of the work by providing extra-premium gas for your child's working muscles. Fat, on the other hand, is used for energy when the sport lasts more than 30 minutes.

FOODS OR SUPPLEMENTS?

If you have a kid who wants you to buy the latest energy supplements at the drug or health food store, teach him to stop believing everything he sees on TV. Supplements won't make jocks stronger or faster. On the other hand, vitamins and minerals are key to helping the body convert food into energy. Athletes (and everyone else) can get vitamins and minerals from eating nutrient-rich foods.

Calcium, for instance, is crucial to athletes because it helps the development of bones. Ever try to run a 100-yard dash with stress fractures? Make sure kids have at least three servings of calcium-rich foods each day. Good calcium sources include low-fat dairy products.

Other minerals are also key players in an athlete's life. Iron deficiencies can lead to poor stamina and some at-risk adolescent girls may have to take supplements. Good sources of iron are meat, fish, and poultry. For a longer list of iron-rich foods, see Chapter 12.

If you introduce kids to pills so early on, they may think the pills, not their own efforts, are making them strong. Or they may become confused when the supplements don't help them. Drill this fact into your kids' heads: Nutritious foods, combined with hard workouts, makes kids big and strong and allows them to become better athletes.

GUZZLE DOWN FOR COMPETITION

Dig out all those promotional water bottles you've brought back from trade shows, fill them up, and put them in your daughter's backpack. She'll need them, because if she is not well-hydrated before, during, and after the game, she may cramp up and collapse on the field.

Water makes up about 60 percent of our body's weight. It serves to move blood, which transfers oxygen to working muscles, and urine, which pushes out metabolic waste products. Most important for your athlete, water regulates her body temperature so she can perspire when she gets too hot.

If your child's organs are practically drowning in water, why should you inundate her with more liquid? Here's why: When your daughter exercises, her working muscles generate heat, which raises her body temperature. Her body gets rid of extra heat by increasing blood flow to the skin and losing heat through ventilation and sweating. The body needs to absorb enough water to keep the cycle going. If she doesn't drink enough water, *dehydration* sets in. Her body heats up, her performance suffers, and her risk of heat injury increases.

WISE WORDS

Dehydration occurs when a person's water content plummets to a dangerously low level. As water is lost through perspiration, the volume of blood goes down, reducing circulation to the skin (and trapping the heat in) and to muscles where nutrients and oxygen are needed. Losing just 2 percent of body weight through perspiration can bring the first signs of dehydration (discomfort, fatigue, headaches). A 5 percent loss leads to heat cramps and heat exhaustion, characterized by a weak, rapid pulse rate and fever. At a 7 percent loss, an athlete may suffer hallucinations, and at a 10 percent loss, she may have a heat stroke.

Pre-adolescents especially need to drink water because their bodies are not well-developed enough to handle temperature extremes. Water is especially crucial if kids are cloaked with sports gear, making it harder for their bodies to sweat, or if swimmers stay out in the sun for long periods waiting for their turn.

Don't wait for your children to ask for water. They won't feel thirsty until well after water loss has occurred. Get your kids to drink both before and during competition, even if they tell you to leave them alone because you are embarrassing them in front of friends.

According to the American Dietetic Association, children should drink the following amounts:

- 10 to 14 ounces of cold water one to two hours before the activity

- 3 to 4 ounces of cold water every 15 minutes during the activity

- 16 ounces of cold water for every pound of weight loss after the exercise

Sports Drinks: Health or Hype?

You often see athletes on TV dumping a cooler of Gatorade over a coach's head. Looks like fun, so kids want it too! These hip, sporty, colorful drinks replace water and electrolytes (sodium, potassium, and chloride) that your kid loses while sweating. Because they contain carbohydrates, sports drinks can give kids extra energy if their games last more than 90 minutes or if competitions take place during intense heat. If your kid refuses to drink water but likes sports drinks, buy one that has 15 to 18 grams of carbohydrates per cup.

If your child is finicky about what he drinks and wants juice only, dilute the stuff to make him happy and keep him hydrated. Mix one cup of water for every cup of juice. Sodas or undiluted juice are out of the question because they are too carbohydrate-heavy and can cause stomach cramps, nausea, and diarrhea. And tell your kid not to stop off at Starbucks on his way to the game. Caffeinated beverages dehydrate the body even more.

Another hydration tip: Give your children watermelon, grapes, and other fruits containing water and carbohydrates. But experts say to never, ever, give salt tablets to your jocks. Athletes can easily replace the sodium they lose to perspiration by eating a healthful diet.

Avoiding Heat Disorders

Heat stroke is the second most common cause of death among high school athletes. Signs of a stroke include: lack of sweat, no urine, dry skin, visual disturbances, fainting, low blood pressure, and shock. If your child gets heat stroke, here's what you should do:

◆ Call for emergency treatment.

◆ Place ice on the back of the child's head.

◆ Remove wet clothing.

◆ If your child is conscious, help him take a cold shower.

◆ If he is in shock, elevate his feet.

In addition to making sure that your young athlete drinks enough fluids, you can take a number of precautions to reduce the risk of heat injury, according to *Play Hard Eat Right, A Parents' Guide to Sports Nutrition for Children* by the American Dietetic Association (1995):

◆ Ask the coach and your child to schedule workouts for the coolest times of the day (before 10 a.m. or after 6 p.m.), particularly in warmer climates.

◆ Allow your child to adjust to warmer weather conditions gradually. Your child and the coach should restrict the length and intensity of training sessions for the first four to five days and then increase the intensity slowly for another one to two weeks.

◆ Don't let your child wear excessive clothing, taping, or padding on hot or humid days. You can help improve body cooling by having him change from sweaty clothes to dry ones. He also should wear white or light-colored clothing made of lightweight cotton or mesh material and low-cut socks.

◆ Make sure the coach schedules breaks in the shade or indoors so that your child's body can cool down.

◆ Make sure that water, preferably chilled water, is available at all times during training and competition.

◆ Make sure that your child comes to practice or competition fully hydrated. Remind him in advance about how much water to drink before arriving.

◆ Weigh your child before and throughout exercise to identify how much weight he loses during practice or competition.

◆ Make sure the coach schedules water breaks during which all children must drink a minimum amount of water.

◆ Pay close attention if your child is at risk for heat disorder due to obesity, poor conditioning, weight loss during exercise, or other health problems.

◆ Discourage the deliberate practice of dehydration. Tell your child that it keeps him from performing up to par athletically and can hurt his body.

◆ Ask the coach to adjust the timing of practice and competition (time of day, season of year) as needed to prevent heat disorders. Extreme heat and/or humidity are valid reasons to cancel a scheduled workout or competition.

BEFORE AND AFTER THE GAME FOODS

Your child has practiced batting for months. The time has come, the big game is tomorrow, and, although he feels ready to take on Roger Clemens, he's nervous. The last thing he needs is to step onto the field an hour after eating at KFC. With all that grease lumped up inside his body, he may feel nauseous, sick to his stomach, and just generally out of sorts. So what should your kids eat before the game? I'll tell you.

Pre-Event Food Preview

The pre-event meal prevents athletes from feeling hungry before or during the event and supplies fuel to the muscles during training and competition. Eating healthfully right before the game won't wipe out the damage done by years of high-fat gorging, but it's a good time to start feeding your athlete well-balanced meals. (Better yet, try feeding her nutritious meals a week before game time.)

Some suggestions for pre-event eating:

♦ Feed your kid three to four hours before the event so the food can be digested. Who wants to have indigestion while they are lunging to head a soccer ball?

♦ Avoid high-fiber foods that will send your child running to a portable toilet instead of second base, and avoid high-fat foods that will weigh her down as she tries to go up for a basket.

♦ Avoid anything high in protein that will take your child too long to digest. Otherwise, she may end up getting nauseated or throwing up—not a pretty sight for the home crowd.

♦ Don't serve your kid beans, broccoli, or other gas-causing foods before the competition.

♦ Keep simple carbohydrates out of your child's reach. Sugar-filled products may taste good, but they won't give her the energy boost she needs to make it through the game.

♦ Serve complex carbohydrates. Fill your child's plate with breads, baked potatoes, pasta with tomato sauce, peanut butter, yogurt, fruit, and other foods rich in carbohydrates.

If the game starts in two to three hours, stay away from dairy products and give your child fruit juices, bagels, and other breads. If you're down to one or two hours before the event, go with fresh fruits and juices for a snack.

Food to Eat at the Game

Some events can last all day, and your kid will be sweltering as he waits his turn. Let him nibble on a carbohydrate snack every 15 to 30 minutes to give him an energy boost. A fig bar, a piece of fruit, or sports drink will do. If your child is on next, he can eat pretzels, muffins, bagels, and sports drinks and stay away from candies, French fries, nachos, and sodas (staple foods at tournaments).

After the Game Feast

The game may be over, but your responsibility toward your child's eating is not. The recovery process, as some call the aftermath of a game, starts as soon as the clapping stops. Start pumping up your kid with carbohydrates and fluids within 30 minutes after exercises. Give her fruit juices while she is putting away her equipment.

Two hours or more after exercising, young jocks should eat a meal of mostly complex carbohydrates, like pasta, breads, fruit, or yogurt. The body is most efficient at absorbing and storing energy during the four to five hours after exercise. These meals are more important because they determine how much energy your young athlete will have for her next training session.

THE LEAST YOU NEED TO KNOW

- ◆ Preteen jocks won't grow bulging muscles until they become sexually mature.

- ◆ Teen jocks must eat more calories, in the form of carbohydrates, than their couch potato peers.

- ◆ Jocks need more proteins than sedentary friends, but too much protein will slow them down in practice sessions and competitions.

- ◆ Athletes should drink 16 ounces of water per each pound lost during exercise to rehydrate.

9

Jump on the Veggie Bandwagon

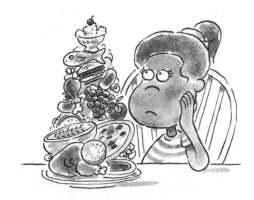

After months of cooking healthful meals, you finally know the food pyramid by heart and can cite the number of servings from each group your kids need. Then, in between picking up your kid from tennis clinic and stopping off at the ATM, one of your children announces: "Mom, I'm becoming a vegetarian."

It may not register right away that all those wonderful chicken dishes you learned to make are no longer useful, or that you'll have to spend more time researching the nutritional values of tofu, tempeh, soy milks, and other products that you still associate with your college food co-op—buckets of bean curds in water, bins of bulgar, bagfuls of stuff you've never heard of.

For years, parents whose kids turned vegetarian have worried about whether their children are getting enough nutrients. Vegetarian diets can be healthful, well-balanced, and enjoyable for everyone if they are well-planned. Vegetarians who eat lots of fruits and vegetables, along with nuts, seeds, and other foods, will get the same nutrients carnivores get from wolfing down meat (if not better). Many vegetarian meals can be made easily and quickly when you get home from work. This chapter focuses on the various types of vegetarians—what they eat and how they can eat right.

HEALTHY VEGETARIAN LIFESTYLES

Why do kids become vegetarians? Many do so for different reasons: some believe it's wrong to kill animals to eat, others feel that processing meats hurts the environment, many cite religious reasons. For many kids, switching to vegetarianism also means adopting a healthier lifestyle. Many vegetarian kids quit smoking and drinking and become interested in nature, volunteer for environmental groups, and become social activists.

A well-planned, balanced vegetarian diet can give your child the nutrients she needs to be healthy. In addition, a well-planned vegetarian diet has the following health benefits:

- ◆ Vegetarians are rarely obese, because their diets consist of mostly plant foods, which have fewer calories and are low in fats (especially saturated fats).

- ◆ Vegetarians tend to have healthier hearts because they have lower blood cholesterol levels.

- ◆ Vegetarians have lower rates of hypertension (abnormally high blood pressure).

- ◆ Vegetarians are at lower risk of osteoporosis, kidney stones, gallstones, and adult-onset diabetes.

But let's not make these guys into nutritional angels either. Some vegetarians can go wild with high-fat cookies, pastas with cream sauces, and other foods. So when you are deciding what to make your vegetarian kids for dinner, keep your eyes on the food pyramid.

VEGETARIAN FOOD GUIDE PYRAMID

Although feeding a vegetarian child is definitely more challenging than feeding a kid who'll eat just about anything (know anyone like that? I don't!), it's not brain surgery. The knowledge you gained from learning the food pyramid in Chapter 2 will come in handy because the vegetarian pyramid (yes, there is one!) is identical for servings of grains, vegetables, fruits, and dairy products.

Instead of the meat group, however, the pyramid features a special vegetarian protein category titled, "Legume, Nut, Seed, and Meat Alternative Group." In this category, the following amounts equal one serving:

◆ Half a cup of cooked beans or peas

◆ Half a cup of tofu

◆ One-quarter of a cup of seeds

◆ One-quarter of a cup (one ounce) of nuts

◆ Two tablespoons of nut butter

◆ One-quarter cup of meat alternative

◆ Two eggs (preferably whites)

Teens who become vegetarians don't have to give up the holy burger roll because they can just stuff them with other meat alternatives, like veggie burgers, soy burgers, and other products. Same deal goes for hot dogs.

ALL IN THE FAMILY

 Seventh-Day Adventists, a religious group whose members advocate vegetarian diets and don't use tobacco or alcohol, have reduced incidences of heart disease. A study reported that 2 percent of this population are vegans, 29 percent are ovolacto-vegetarians, 25 percent eat meat once a week, 29 percent eat meat one to four times a week, and 15 percent eat meat five or more times a week. Is their rate of heart disease reduced because of their low-meat diet or healthy lifestyle? Nobody knows for sure.

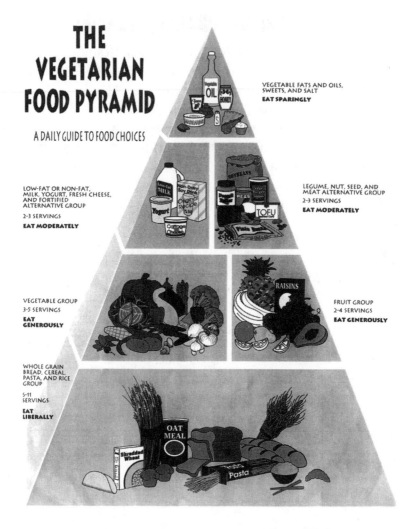

The Vegetarian Food Pyramid: A Daily Guide To Food Choices © from The Health Connection, 1-800-548-8700. You can order posters or handouts by calling (301) 790-9735.

Follow this guide carefully to make sure your kids get all the nutrients they need to flourish as vegetarians.

SEMIS, LACTOS, VEGANS: MEET TODAY'S VEGETARIANS

Thought you were hip just because you have vegetarian friends and ate tofu once? If all vegetarians seem the same to you, you've been living in a food warp. Just being a plain old vegetarian is old hat. Here are the four main categories of vegetarians, based on what they will and will not eat:

◆ **Vegans** These vegetarians are the purest, holier-than-thou vegetarians. They won't eat any animal products, including eggs or dairy. Their basic diet is plant food products: grains, legumes, fruits, vegetables, nuts, and seeds. Only two percent of all American vegetarians are vegans.

◆ **Lacto-vegetarians** In addition to not eating any meat, poultry, fish, or seafood, these vegetarians also eliminate eggs and egg products from their diets. They will eat all dairy products, though.

◆ **Ovolacto-vegetarians** This category of vegetarians won't eat meat, poultry, fish and seafood, but they eat dairy products and eggs.

◆ **Semi-vegetarians** This group doesn't eat red meat, but they do eat chicken or fish once in a while. Semi-vegetarians also eat dairy products and eggs.

In case you aren't confused enough already, many other vegetarian variations exist. Your kid wants to eat fish, but not meat or chicken? He can join the *pesco-vegetarians*. If your daughter prefers chicken, but not fish or red meat, she is a *pollo-vegetarian*.

Some people also eliminate certain foods because of the way they are prepared or because they contain certain chemicals or other substances. Some people only eat organically grown foods, others only consume raw plants, and a few (called *fruitarians*) eat only fruit, nuts, seeds, honey, olive oil, and whole grains.

BEST VERY VEGGIE MEALS

Whether your child is an ovolacto, lacto, or pesco vegetarian—it's tough to remember what's what—you will have to plan meals extra carefully to ensure he gets all the necessary nutrients. First, read up about vegetarian nutrition (this book is a good start), then plan a vegetarian menu that includes all the nutrients your child needs to sprout (just a joke).

It's not as hard as you think.

Vying for Protein

Most of us get our fill of proteins without blinking an eye. Grams tally up as we eat our morning eggs (cholesterol-free, I hope!), turkey sandwiches at lunch, and fish or chicken entree at dinner. Protein is also found in plants, but, as mentioned in Chapter 2, no one plant food supplies all the amino acids necessary for growth.

The key in feeding your vegetarian child (if she eats little or no meat, fish, or poultry) a balanced diet is to put together two plant foods that contain complementary amino acids so that combined, they give your child their best protein power. For instance, cereal grains (wheat) are poor in the essential amino acid *lysine*, but they are rich in *methionine*. Legumes (dried peas and beans), on the other hand, provide enough lysine but little methionine. Mixing grains and legumes, then, gives your child a powerhouse combination.

WISE WORDS

Tofu is soy protein made from soy milk curds that you can use to make practically any dish you want. Tofu comes in three forms: firm, soft, and silken. Because tofu is basically flavorless, it takes on the flavor of whatever else you've got in the pot. Throw tofu in the wok with vegetables, make soups with it, puree it in pies, or chuck it in salads, and your child will have a healthful entree.

Vitamin B12: Gotta Have It

Vegetarians need only a tad of vitamin B12, but they probably won't get it unless they eat eggs and milk products. A main player in the formation of red blood cells, B12 is also found in algae, spirulina, and fermented products (Yuck!), but these products aren't for human consumption. Most vegetarians must consume foods fortified with B12. These foods include the following:

- Fortified soy milk, milk substitutes
- Cereals
- Nutritional yeast

Check with your doctor or dietitian about whether your child should be taking B12 supplements. It takes a long time for a B12 deficiency to show up, but the effects can be as bad as severe anemia and irreversible neurological damage.

Mock Milk

Vegetarians who avoid dairy products may have a tough time meeting calcium requirements. Dairy products provide about three-fourths of the calcium in our diets, but fruits and veggies provide only one-tenth of what we need. Your child needs calcium to build her bones and teeth and help other parts of her body function properly. Here are some calcium alternatives:

- Fortified soy milk products (tofu, soybean, tempeh)
- Dark green leafy vegetables (collard greens, broccoli)
- Molasses
- Calcium-fortified grains
- Calcium-fortified orange juice
- Supplements

If your vegetarian child is not an extremist, you'll have to keep an eye on what he eats, but you won't have to stand over him. If your child is a true-blue vegan, you have some work to do. You can probably find most mock-milk products in a regular supermarket. But you may have to haunt health-food stores and supermarkets to get a product fortified with B12 vitamins.

But it's worth the extra effort. Your child's health depends on it.

Pumping Iron

Non-vegetarians get plenty of iron from red meats, chicken, eggs, and many other products. But vegetarian diets can be low in iron—a nutrient that carries oxygen in the red-blood cells—if not properly planned. So what's a mom to do? Get your kid to eat other iron-rich foods:

- Dried beans

- Spinach

- Bulgar

- Prune juice

- Dried fruits

- Blackstrap molasses

- Enriched and whole-grain breads

- Wheat germ

- Seeds, nuts

- Potato skins

- Tofu, miso

- Brewer's yeast

- Fortified cereals

MOM KNOWS BEST

 Because iron from plant foods isn't as easily absorbed as iron from animal foods, serve your vegetarian foods that are high in Vitamin C at each meal. Vitamin C boosts iron absorption.

Kids Need Zinc to Be in Sync

Zinc, a mineral essential to the function of more than 70 enzymes in the body, is found in seafood, meats, and eggs. Vegetarians get some zinc from plant sources, but because plant zinc doesn't get absorbed by the body very well, vegetarian children need to make sure they eat plenty of plant foods that are rich in zinc:

- Nuts

- Legumes

- Miso

◆ Pumpkin and sunflower seeds

◆ Whole-grain yeast breads

◆ Tofu

◆ Wheat germ

Did you ever think there were so many foods you'd never heard of? Most of us have been confined to supermarket shopping for years and never noticed anything other than the stuff we come in to buy. So welcome to the world of vegetarian foods!

INTRO TO VEGAN NUTRITION

Feeding most semi-vegetarians is virtually no problem, especially if your family already eats chicken or fish. But preparing meals for vegans is an entirely different challenge, because you'll have to start preparing foods that you may not know very much about, if anything at all.

Because the vegan diet is so restrictive, nearly everybody who is anybody in the mainstream medical field expresses concerns about its hazards for young children. If your child is on a vegan diet, experts suggest that he be routinely monitored by a pediatrician who will work with a dietitian to assure normal growth and development.

11 MEALS FOR VEGETARIANS

When you come home after all-day meetings, it's hard enough to think about what to cook with ingredients you've used all your life. Off the top of your head, could you come up with any ideas for what to feed your vegan child? Most of us can't. So we rely on others to do the thinking for us.

Sharon K. Yntema's book *Vegetarian Children, A Supportive Guide For Parents* (McBooks Press, 1987) gives some great ideas for foods you can feed your vegetarian child:

◆ Ramen noodles with tofu chunks and peas as soup or casserole. But be careful, the noodles are high in fat.

- Macaroni and cheese and peas (any noodles with cheese sauce)

- Oatmeal with wheat germ, raisins, and cinnamon

- Pasta (spaghetti or any whole-grain pasta) and tomato sauce (add well-cooked soy grits for extra flavor and nutrition)

- Cottage cheese with peas and a whole-grain bread with a nut spread

- Vegetarian burgers or patties with whole-grain roll, catsup, and salad

- Rice and nuts or seeds with vegetable side dishes

- Pizza (whole-grain crust spread with tomato puree, oregano, and cheese)

- Scrambled tofu (Mash tofu to scrambled egg-like consistency. Mix with egg or a little tahini and a dash of soy sauce or cheese. Cook like scrambled eggs.)

- Whole-grain pancakes with grated vegetables in the batter, served with applesauce or sour cream

- Potato pancakes with wheat germ

For more vegetarian recipes, get a copy of *The New Laurel's Kitchen* by Laurel Robertson, which is an excellent vegetarian cookbook and reference.

ALL IN THE FAMILY

Add soy food—a type of protein that comes in many forms—to any meal, and you'll boost your child's protein intake without the high fat and extra calories that typically go along with meat consumption. Can't go wrong with that! A half cup of soy flour, for example, (used in quick breads, muffins and other products) supplies 22 grams of protein. Isolated soy protein, a powdery substance that's 90 percent pure protein, can be used in pancakes, cereals, pasta, soups, and sauces. A one-ounce serving yields between 13 to 23 grams of protein. Other types of soy foods include soymilk, tempeh, tofu, and other variations.

DEALING WITH VEGETARIAN CHILDREN

If everyone at home is a vegetarian, dinner times should be smooth sailing. But what happens when your child is the only vegetarian, and he sees his calling as imposing vegetarian values on earth, starting with his own family? Here are some tips on how to deal with vegetarian crusaders:

◆ Don't let your child become a food tyrant. If he calls you an animal killer as you are about to take a bite of your chicken, tell him that just as you respect him for choosing to be a vegetarian, you expect him to respect you for your dietary choices. If he continues being obnoxious, tell him you won't tolerate that behavior and that he'll be asked to sit someplace else at dinner so he doesn't disrupt everyone else's meal.

◆ If your child gripes that your vegetarian meals are "boring," remind him that the choice to become a vegetarian was his, not yours. Say that you'd be happy to take some vegetarian cookbooks out of the library so both you and he can look at the recipes and decide what you can both, or he alone, can cook. (If he expects you to do it all, tell him he isn't really committed to being a vegetarian.)

◆ If he complains that the food at the supermarket isn't "organic" enough for him and he'd like you to drive out to the co-op eight miles away from home, decide whether you are willing to take him to the co-op. If you can't afford organic foods (they are more expensive), just tell him outright. If you don't feel like schlepping him out there, help him find a ride or give him a bus schedule.

◆ Don't bother cooking two meals all the time just because you and your son want something different. Find neutral entrees where you both get, say, pasta with veggies. You can toss chicken on your dish, while he enjoys the meat-less entree. This is less work and everyone walks away a little happier. (But don't expect your child to be too grateful.)

◆ Warn your child about having an "attitude" when your family goes out to eat and she sees animals served on a plate. Tell her that she can have a vegetarian option, if one exists. If there is no special item on the menu, then she can have salads, side dishes of veggies, or just make do with other non-meat alternatives. If worse comes to worse, she can order a salad sandwich.

◆ If your child is going to a barbecue, assure her that she won't starve there. Pack up some veggie burgers (you can buy them in the frozen food section of most supermarkets) in her backpack along with tofu dogs and tell her to throw them on the grill. Once it's in the hamburger bun, nobody will notice the difference. Plus, she'll probably run into many takers.

THE LEAST YOU NEED TO KNOW

◆ Vegetarians range from people who just avoid red meat to those who refuse to eat any animal products, including eggs and dairy.

◆ Vegetarian diets are healthier because they tend to be low in saturated fats.

◆ The vegetarian food pyramid emphasizes legumes, nuts, seeds, and other protein sources as alternatives to meats.

◆ Vegan diets require careful planning with the help of a nutritionist.

◆ Support your child's vegetarianism, but don't let him control the rest of the family's food choices. But be cautious. Vegan diets require careful planning to prevent inadequate nutrition. If you need help in developing a balanced diet, contact a nutritionist.

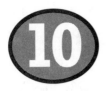

Childhood Obesity: A Major American Problem

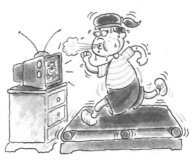

In This Chapter

- ◆ Why the number of obese American kids is on the rise
- ◆ Fattening combo: Too much TV, too little exercise
- ◆ Is your child obese?
- ◆ Feeding your chubby child
- ◆ What to say to your overweight child

Many of us feel anxious when our children get chubby. We worry that they'll be ridiculed, that nobody will want to play with them, and that they'll be lonely and depressed and suffer from low self-esteem. Your chubby child may feel OK about her weight, but your anxiety about her weight, and any restrictive diet you put her on, sends her the message that she is not OK the way she is. This approach may make her eat more (or not eat) to spite you.

Many experts say you shouldn't put obese adolescents on rigid, restrictive diets. Instead, you should feed them what you should be feeding all your kids: low-fat balanced meals filled with grains, vegetables, and fruits. Nutritious meals, lots of exercise, and regularly scheduled healthful snacks will help slim down your kid and establish good eating patterns for her future. The key is to focus on nutrition, not calories, although you should also try serving smaller portions without making a big fuss. You could also serve high-calorie foods less often so your child doesn't feel deprived—or punished for being overweight.

In this chapter, I define obesity, explain why so many kids are overweight, and tell you what you can do to help your children slim down without creating huge battles that ultimately make your kids feel worse.

OBESITY: AMERICA'S TOP NUTRITIONAL DISORDER

Obesity is the most common nutritional disorder in American children; it affects between 10 to 25 percent of kids today. Studies show that as many as 11 million children between ages 6 and 17 may be overweight, and they are getting heavier with each generation. An average 10-year-old child today is 3.5 pounds heavier than the average 10-year-old child of 15 years ago. Once kids are obese, it's hard to get them to trim down. Obese adolescents have only a 1 in 28 chance of becoming normal-weight adults.

WISE WORDS

How do docs determine if your child has a weight problem? Typically, they glance at a standard height/weight chart and see where your child fits into the normal range. He is deemed:

◆ Overweight, if his weight is 10 to 20 percent higher than normal

◆ Obese, if he is 20 percent or more above normal weight

◆ Morbidly obese, if his weight is 50 to 100 percent over normal weight.

But some docs think these charts are based on the wrong criteria, according to the *PDR Family Guide to Nutrition and Health* (Medical Economics Company, 1995). The guide says that some people ditch the chart and look for the following signals to see if their child needs to change his eating patterns:

◆ Does your kid feel energetic or tired all the time? Can he go up the stairs without stopping to catch his breath?

◆ Does his back hurt or does he have any health problems like diabetes or high blood pressure?

◆ Can you pinch an inch of fat at his waist or behind his arm?

◆ What is his overall muscle tone? Flabby or firm?

◆ Has his pediatrician said he needs to be better fit?

According to some pediatricians, school-age kids establish their eating patterns and don't like to change them. Yet, continuing to let them eat high-fat foods excessively—or just overeat healthful foods—can be dangerous. Here is why:

◆ Overweight adolescents are at higher risk for future heart disease.

◆ Overweight adolescents can have respiratory problems.

◆ Overweight adolescents have orthopedic difficulties caused by the extra weight placed on their joints.

◆ The National Institutes of Health (NIH) declared obesity a "biologic hazard" that should be treated as aggressively as any other disease. The NIH says that at least 40 percent of all cases of high blood pressure could be prevented by controlling weight.

Overeating, eating unhealthful foods, and lack of exercise are the major causes of obesity. It's difficult for some parents to admit that their child is obese or gaining weight so rapidly that she's heading down that path. But to really help their child, parents must attack the weight problem head on and find out what they can do to change their child's eating habits.

WHAT CAUSES OBESITY?

Children become overweight when they take in more calories than their bodies can burn. The extra calories get stored as fat. Some accumulation of fat in existing *adipocytes* (fat cells) is normal, especially in girls undergoing puberty. Pre-adolescent boys "pudge out" too. But obese adolescents produce many new adipocytes as well, above and beyond what their bodies need.

The really bad news about adipocytes is that once your child reaches adulthood, the number of fat cells accumulate and become permanent residents in his body. They can't be decreased or increased. They can be shrunk by dieting, but the kid is stuck with the fat cells forever—cells that wait with bated breath to digest any fat that comes down the pipe.

Blame It on the Tube

Some kids become overweight by sitting too many hours in front of the tube, gorging themselves with chips and other high-fat snacks, and not budging unless the pizza delivery guy arrives. As soon as your son comes home from school to an empty house, what does he do? He gets himself a snack, and then watches TV. What does he see? Commercials for fast food, sugary cereals, and cookies, and beverages (sodas, Kool-Aid)—all of which are high in calories and God knows how many fats.

ALL IN THE FAMILY

 At an American Heart Association conference last year, one expert nutritionist reported that in 1993, commercials for high-fat foods made up 41 percent of total commercials shown on Saturday morning, as compared to 16 percent in 1990. Researchers have found that for each hour your kid spends watching TV, he becomes 2 percent less active—and closer to obesity.

TV turns your kids into loafers and junk food connoisseurs. Consider these facts:

◆ A kid between 6 and 11 years old may watch an average of 24 hours of TV a week; that's equivalent to two to three full-time days at your office!

◆ Watching more than 12 hours of TV a week has been shown to have a negative effect on school performance.

What obese children need, in addition to a nutritional tune-up, is exercise. Unless he is willing to take the tube on a bike ride or walk, suggest he turn off the television and get some exercise.

Blame It on Lethargy

If you are handing the remote control to your kid after she gets home from school, figuring she needs a rest from shooting hoops in gym, you've got your facts wrong. Most of us remember physical education: swimming, tennis, floor exercises (Yuck, I still recall when they measured our waists!), but physical education isn't what it used to be. Some elementary schoolchildren only have 25 minutes of physical activity a week; others have less. Others only need one year of physical education to graduate from high school. And, even more frightening, many private schools don't even have physical education teachers for elementary grades.

When physical activity *is* offered, the focus is more on learning the sport and beating the other team than on health. Because overweight children often don't move as fast, they get turned off to sports. (I still feel a tinge of pain when recalling that old Janis Ian song about being the last one picked for basketball.) Obese kids—like all kids—can benefit from aerobic exercise that anyone can do at any pace, but kids in this age group do not view aerobic exercise as being cool. Riding their bikes, playing hide and go seek, and chasing you will get their bodies moving. And that's definitely more cool that riding a stationary bike that goes nowhere.

Blame It on the Genes

Obesity can be inherited within families. If parents are overweight, their kids will likely be overweight as well. Look at the following facts:

- If one parent is overweight, statistics show a 40 percent chance that at least one child will be fat.
- If both parents tip the scale, the chance for an overweight kid increases to 80 percent.

Genetic factors determine when your child has eaten enough, where fat is stored in his body, and how long his body takes to burn calories. But just because the genes for obesity get passed down doesn't mean your child is doomed to be overweight. The problem is that many parents assume their kids will follow in their footsteps.

After dozens of failed crash diets, weight-loss programs, and other frustrating efforts, many parents just say, "What's the point?" They file into their minivan and go to Burger King, where they gulp down more calories from cheeseburgers, french fries, and chocolate shakes, perpetuating greasy food values to their kids.

Although genes do make your children vulnerable to heaviness, what they eat, how much they eat, and how active they are carries a lot of weight (no pun intended). The child prone to obesity always comes up against the genetic struggle to keep fit, but this battle can be won. The best time to teach your children how to live a healthful life and start them on a well-balanced diet is now. And for it to work, it's helpful when the entire family eats a well-balanced diet as well.

Blame It on a Tough Life

Kids with personal or family problems can also become overweight. *Emotional overeating*—when a child disregards hunger cues and eats when she is sad, angry, stressed, or bored—also contributes to weight gain. Some emotional problems get so bad that children may develop an eating disorder, digging themselves deeper and deeper into the weight-loss war. (See Chapter 11 on eating disorders.)

ARE YOU OBSESSED WITH YOUR CHILD'S WEIGHT?

When your child was an infant, remember how you fretted over her weight? "Can you believe I pushed this 10-pounder out?" you said to your friends, beaming with pride. "I'm sure he'll grow," you may have said to people, lowering your voice to explain the low birth weight of your baby. Funny that by the time kids get to be adolescents, we worry that they're too heavy!

Mothers, especially those who have battled extra weight all their lives, panic when their kids start looking chunkier. They put their kids on restrictive diets, glaring at them when they take an extra serving of gravy and scowling every time they reach for another cookie. But denying children food often backfires because they end up wanting to eat more. Often this type of obsessive atmosphere creates eating disorders.

A friend told me that her daughter's classmate, a chubby child whose mother is constantly telling her not to eat this and that, once dumped an entire broccoli platter on her plate as food was being passed around at dinner. "I was glad she was eating something healthy," my friend said, "but the way she did it was disturbing. She needed to hoard everything." Her mother, it turns out, limited what she could eat at dinner—even the good stuff!

If you are the kind of person who overreacts to food issues, examine your own attitudes about weight and diet before imposing your eating style on your child. The last thing you want to do is make your child think that being thin is ideal. This message will surely upset her and trigger a lifetime of eating problems.

At the other extreme are mothers who don't care what their overweight kids eat (or don't know any better) and make no attempts to ensure their children grow up with healthy eating patterns. These mothers pass on the impression that every food is just as good as any other food and give their children total freedom to choose anything.

For these kids to thrive, both mother and child need nutrition education so that they can change their mindsets about eating and health. Parents like these may need the help of a dietitian to learn what children should eat, as well as a psychotherapist to talk over emotional issues revolving around food. These are the types of questions that may come up in counseling:

- Is food served at home as a reward for doing well in school?

- Do parents give kids ice cream to cheer them up when they are down?

- Is dessert withheld until the child cleans her plate?

- Is dessert always junk food, or is fruit often served instead?

It's painful to see how many of our own weight problems resurface as we deal with our children's' weight. But we now know that our children will pay a high price for being grossly overweight—heart disease. We must help them, and the best thing we can do for them is to teach them to eat healthfully. And, in the process, teach ourselves the same thing.

HOW MUCH SHOULD YOUR KIDS WEIGH?

Before you decide whether your child has a weight problem, consider these facts:

◆ Normal bodies come in different sizes and shapes.

◆ Kids the same age grow at different rates.

◆ It's normal for preteen girls to gain weight and for their bodies to look more rounded as they enter puberty. Boys also go through their own changes as they become more sexually mature.

◆ An increase in height is usually accompanied by weight gain.

To make sure you are not projecting your own fat fears on your child, get an outside opinion. Ask your pediatrician: Is my child overweight or not? If so, what can I do to help him reach the right weight? Your pediatrician will check how your child is growing by tracking his height and weight on a standardized growth chart (a chart that covers the range of weights and heights of other Americans the same age and sex). The best thing about getting a chart reading is that it's objective, untainted by your fears and projections; this information lets you know where your child stands in the overall picture. If your child falls between the 5th and 95 percentile for weight, he's fine.

If over a period of time, your child has shifted more than two percentile groups for weight (from, say, the 50th to 90th percentile), then further evaluation may be needed, according to the *Yale Guide To Children's Nutrition* (Yale University, 1997). If his weight drops to a much lower percentage, something may be wrong medically.

MOM KNOWS BEST

Before you declare your child overweight, think about your own ideas about body images and then decide whether you should pass them on to your children. Young children are already weight-conscious. One study found that 45 percent of boys and girls in grades three to six wanted to be thinner and 37 percent tried to lose weight. Many of them said they wanted to be thin because parents and friends always wanted to be skinny.

GETTING YOUR CHILD IN SHAPE

To help your obese children get in shape, you need to get more involved in their lives. So put down your briefcase and go for a walk with them. Speak to your pediatrician about whether to enroll your child in a weight-loss class—but be careful. You don't want to make a big issue out of your child's weight. You do, however, want to make a big deal out of eating nutritious, balanced meals.

Take Control: Seize the Remote

How do you yank the remote control away from your child's hands? Set times for viewing and enforce a limit on the number of hours of TV watching per day. Teach your children some critical viewing skills; for example, explain that TV commercials show only the positive aspect of a product, not the negative.

What if nobody is home when your kids get home from school? Urge your kids to get out of the house to exercise, go to a friend's house, or go to the park. Another option is to sign them up for after-school activities to keep them active and preoccupied. The Y has terrific after-school programs for kids of all ages. Also, make sure you plan activities for your children during the summer. Encourage them to volunteer, go on nature hikes, and do other activities. The more engaged they are in an activity, the less likely they'll be to think about eating.

Get Your Child Up and At It

Your child has to get more exercise if he is to beat obesity. Physical activity reduces fat, helps the heart stay in shape, gives children a feeling of accomplishment, and is just plain fun. Because most obese adolescents will be engaged in lifelong weight battles, the best activities for them are those they can do for the rest of their lives either alone or with others. These activities include the following:

◆ Tennis

◆ Swimming

◆ Skating

◆ Dancing (they can do it in their own living room!)

◆ Walking

Exercising is fun for the whole family. There are lots of fun, easy activities you can enjoy with your overweight child that will bring the family closer together. When you play sports with him, remember to always cheer for him, give him a pat on the back for good effort, and be light on criticism. The goal is not to score, but to get him to play.

Here are some ideas for family exercises:

◆ Go for evening walks after dinner.

◆ Put in an exercise video and get the family to stretch, do sit-ups, and leg raises. Kids always have fun watching mom and dad be clumsy.

◆ Go on bike rides.

◆ Take a hike with a healthy picnic lunch and plenty of water.

◆ Sign up for family in-line skating lessons.

◆ Swim laps together (build up the number gradually).

◆ Play volleyball at the beach.

◆ Join a soccer, t-ball, or other sport league.

The point is, do something—anything! And it's up to you to set the example. Do it for your child, and do it for yourself. If you instill the right philosophy in your child, you're helping to ensure that she'll do the same for your grandchildren someday!

CUT BACK ON FAT

When adults go on a diet, they cut back on calories, but with kids dieting is more complicated. Regardless of whether they are obese, kids need calories to grow. They also need a diet that provides the necessary balance of carbos, protein, and fats, as well as plenty of fruits and vegetables. Most experts say that restrictive diets at this stage are no-nos. Teenagers consuming 1,800 calories or less may not meet requirements for nutrients like calcium, iron, zinc, and vitamins A and C.

Plus, saying no to your children all the time will make them mad and rebellious—not a good combination. You don't have to play the role of food cop all the time. Instead of withholding food, structure their eating schedules so they can eat smaller portions at meals and snacks instead. This approach, along with exercise and counseling (if your kids have emotional or social problems), will help your kids lose weight without feeling deprived. Also, teach kids to make choices—give them a list of nutritious snacks and let them decide what they want to eat.

Ask your doctor whether your children need to lose weight or maintain their weight while they grow into the right body proportions over time. If they have to maintain their weight, make sure they are burning off the same number of calories that they are taking in—otherwise, the extra calories will get stored as fat. One way to check whether your child is maintaining his weight is to weigh him. What a brilliant idea! If he has to lose weight, you may need to be more structured about feeding him. (See "Dealing with Your Chubby Child," later in this chapter, for tips.)

Be practical and flexible and work with your child when you are designing a menu. Always emphasize more exercise rather than less food. Make sure you give your children a variety of foods to choose from and the right number of calories for their age, size, and energy level. Examine your children's eating patterns and determine whether they need to change. To treat obesity, look at the following issues:

◆ On average, does the kid eat the right amount of food based on his energy requirements?

◆ When does your child eat the most? At meals or in between?

◆ Is he drinking too many high-calorie beverages?

◆ Is there a relationship between when she eats and what she is doing?

◆ Is she moving around? Playing sports?

◆ Is there a relationship between her eating habits and her emotions?

Keep a journal of how your kids are doing once treatment starts. Then look over your notes and talk to your doctor about which habits need to be changed. Target one of these habits, such as eating between meals. If your child snacks between meals (which she should), divide the day's menu into small meals throughout the day rather than restricting food to three big meals. Scheduling healthful snacks helps kids get the extra calories they need and is a good, legitimate way for obese kids to eat low-fat foods without having to "cheat." (For more details on regulating snacks, see Chapter 7.)

Scheduling healthful snacks helps kids get the extra calories they need and is a good, legitimate way for obese kids to eat low-fat foods. But don't be a spoilsport. Let them go for the high-lead stuff once in a while—and give them a limit on, say, 100 to 150 calories. You can make them a list of foods falling into that range, and have them choose their favorite.

To keep tabs on where your child's calories are coming from, keep a diary of what he eats during a week. He'll have to help you record what he consumes when you aren't with him. Were most of his meals hamburgers, french fries, and hot dogs? Did he drink lots of high-calorie beverages? Did he eat three large bowls of cereal with milk as a snack?

The message you want to pass on to your child regarding junk food is this: "Have less of it, less often." You also want to teach your child the importance of appropriate portions. Start off with this simple rule: Only one high calorie/high-fat food a day and tell your child, "If you eat french fries, you don't get cake."

DEALING WITH YOUR CHUBBY CHILD

To help your obese child become more fit, don't deprive him of all the food he used to like. What you are trying to do is teach him to follow his inner cues about hunger and fullness so that he'll be able to regulate when to eat and when to stop on his own some day. Keep these pointers in mind when dealing with your overweight child:

◆ Don't get rid of all the stuff he likes to eat at once (others in the house might resent it too!). Gradually introduce good nutritional foods into your cooking. These slow changes will help the entire family adapt to a new way of eating, so the child who brought on this change in first place isn't blamed for putting everyone on a diet.

- Treat your chubby child like everyone else in the family with respect to food. If you want him to eat an apple, don't give everyone else chocolate cake a la mode. Serve everyone a treat, and emphasize portion control for everyone.

- Keep a healthy feeding relationship, says Ellyn Satter in *How To Get Your Kid To Eat...But Not Too Much*. You are responsible for what is available for your child to eat, and he is responsible for how much he eats. When you are serving healthful meals, your kids should be able to have as much as they want.

- Maintain the structure of meals and snacks, Satter suggests. This way, your overweight child knows that he'll get enough to eat throughout the day, so he doesn't have to scarf down everything on his plate during the meal, afraid that nothing else will be offered until dinner.

- Encourage your child to be active, but don't tell him that he is lazy and needs to exercise if he wants to look decent. Rather, let him know that his sedentary style is common; a study showed that ⅔ of our youth between ages 6 to 17 couldn't pass a basic fitness test. Exercise is the best thing he can do. Try to set goals for swimming *x* number of laps in the pool or walking for *x* number of minutes, so your child can have a feeling of accomplishment.

- Your child will be more likely to make changes if he knows that you love him no matter what.

- Emphasize fitness, not fatness.

- Don't feed your child unnecessarily, Satter adds. Don't reward your overweight child (or any child) with a piece of cake when he hurts his knee. Don't give soft drinks or juice when water will do. All of these "rewards" add extra calories to your child's diet—calories that may show up later as fat.

- Most importantly, set a good example! Follow good eating habits yourself.

THE LEAST YOU NEED TO KNOW

◆ Between 10 to 25 percent of kids today are considered obese.

◆ Watching too much TV, not getting enough exercise, genetic makeup, or depression can set up a child for obesity.

◆ Parents should confirm their child's obesity with a doctor. Children should fall within the 5 to 95 percentile for weight for their height.

◆ Get your kids in shape by limiting TV, encouraging more exercise, and serving healthful foods.

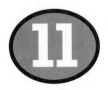

Eating Disorders

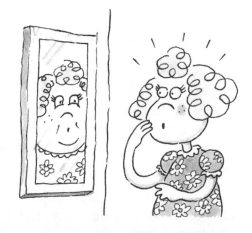

You look at your bright, confident, fun-loving daughter who has just been diagnosed with anorexia nervosa, and you scratch your head. Why? Or you hear that your friend repeatedly catches her daughter, the best gymnast in the school, in the bathroom throwing up whatever she just ate.

Statistics show that as many as 10 to 15 percent of adolescent girls and young women in the U.S. suffer from eating disorders. A small percentage of boys are also afflicted. Some starve themselves, others binge and purge, and many just eat too much. A large number don't meet the criteria to be full-blown anorexics or bulimics, but their eating patterns are leading them in that direction.

Check out the following statistics from Eating Disorders Awareness and Prevention, Inc.:

◆ Between 1 and 3 percent of middle school and high school girls become bulimic.

◆ Between .25 percent and 1 percent of middle school and high school girls become anorexic.

◆ Between 2 to 13 percent of middle school and high school girls have *atypical eating disorder*, a food disorder that could mark the beginning of anorexia or bulimia.

This chapter gives you background on the different types of eating disorders, how to feed children suffering from these diseases, and what to do to help prevent children from using food to cover up deeper feelings.

THIN IS IN

Many preteens and teens aspire to be like the glamorous women portrayed in magazines, TV, and advertising. Raised in a weight-conscious society, your daughter, like many of us, may believe that being skinny is the key to happiness, success, and beauty. Imagine the pressure she must withstand in trying to reach that ideal when her body is beginning to mature sexually. It's hard to compete with paper-thin movie stars or models when she feels squeamish about her developing breasts and horrified by the newly rounded body shape she is acquiring. So what does she do? Hold on to her innocence. How? By starving herself to stay small and stave off the awkward feelings of becoming a woman.

Not all girls are vulnerable to eating disorders; girls who develop food disorders tend to have low self-esteem and depend on others for decisions and approval. Most also have underlying family conflicts. They think, "If I could just be thin, my life would change and I'd be great, successful, attractive, and in control of things." Their bodies are going through a growth spurt but many of them don't realize that they have to eat more to meet their bodies' needs. They are afraid that eating more will make them obese.

Kids with eating disorders are in trouble and they need professional help: help to get medically back on track, to deal with the causes of their food obsession, and to develop healthy eating patterns to lead the rest of their lives.

WISE WORDS

An eating disorder, says Ellyn Satter, author of *How To Get Your Kid To Eat...But Not Too Much,* is not the same thing as an eating problem. An eating problem starts when families who want their kids to eat well run up against finicky eaters. An eating disorder, however, develops when families ignore their children's eating problems until one of them becomes anorexic or bulimic. Then everyone should go into treatment, because family problems must be worked out before the eating struggles stop.

ANOREXIA NERVOSA: DYING TO BE THIN

Anorexia nervosa is a psychological disorder characterized by self-induced starvation. Girls who suffer from this disorder think they are overweight, even though they may be thin as a rail. Because they are starving themselves, girls with this disorder suffer nutritional deficiencies that can have devastating effects on their health.

WISE WORDS

Anorexia nervosa is an eating disorder that hits most girls during the teen years (sometimes even earlier). Girls and women afflicted with it refuse to eat, and lose so much weight that they jeopardize their physical and psychological well-being.

Symptoms and Effects of Anorexia

According to Eating Disorders Awareness and Prevention, Inc. (EDAP), anorexia affects .25 to one percent of middle and high school girls. It's estimated that up to 50 percent of girls with anorexia eventually become bulimic.

- Anorexics often lose more than 25 percent of their body weight and can get down to as little as 70 pounds. To keep the brain and heart going, the body slows down other vital processes, so the thyroid function is reduced, the blood pressure drops, and the heart rate lowers.

- Anorexia causes dry skin, hair loss, and constipation.

- *Amenorrhea*, the inability to menstruate, is a major diagnostic symptom of anorexia. Girls need a certain percentage of body fat to gear up for the menstrual cycle. In about 30 percent of all anorexics, the period stops before there has been substantial weight loss.

- Loss of bone mass due to *osteoporosis*, a condition in which bones lose mass and become fragile or brittle, is another physical symptom of anorexia. Not all women will recover lost bone mass when they get back to their normal weight, so they'll be more likely to get wrist, hip, and vertebrae fractures after menopause.

- Anorexics also experience mild *anemia*—a deficiency in the number of red blood cells resulting in swelling of joints, difficulty sleeping, and reduced muscle mass. Like bulimics—who gorge themselves with food and then get rid of it through vomiting or using laxatives—anorexics may also binge and purge.

These facts are pretty scary. Your child could die because of some emotional problem you may or may not be aware of and in pursuit of a beauty standard that, when reached, delivers only disappointment. But you can help your child overcome this disease. Once your anorexic daughter gets back to normal eating, she'll probably regain her health. However, sometimes the damage is so severe that even normal eating won't help. Remember Karen Carpenter? She suffered heart failure just months after she started eating normally. That's why it's important to pay close attention to your child's eating habits and weight and act quickly at the first signs of a problem.

Early Signs of Anorexia

Your life is so busy that you may often feel like you can't see what's right in front of your face, including your daughter rapidly losing weight. But you must open your eyes to anorexia nervosa if you want to catch the disease in its early stages. The following signs should raise red flags:

- Your daughter's eating changes drastically from day to day. For example, she may eat nothing one day and clean the plate the next.

- Your daughter appears to be obsessed with dieting.

- Your daughter loses 15 percent or more of her normal body weight because she is depriving herself of calories.

- Your daughter weighs herself constantly and exercises excessively.

- Your daughter always refers to herself as being chunky or having a bulging stomach or fat thighs, even though she appears normal.

- Your daughter constantly thinks about food, but refuses to eat.

- Your daughter develops dry skin and hair, skin rashes, and is sluggish.

- Your daughter acts depressed and withdrawn.

- Your daughter misses at least three consecutive periods.

If you think your daughter is suffering from anorexia, don't reason with her or force her to eat. And don't wait! First, take her to an MD for evaluation. If the disorder is severe, your doctor may suggest she undergo treatment that involves a dietitian, a medical doctor, and psychiatrist. If you're lucky enough to perceive that your daughter has an eating disorder before it gets really bad, take her for an evaluation right away and find out what steps to take so she can get back on track—both nutritionally and psychologically.

BULIMIA: THE BINGE/PURGE SYNDROME

Remember in college when friends would "pig out" at the dinning commons and come back to the dorm to throw up? Many of us thought "bingeing and barfing" was just a passing phase, one of those "college things." Although news blared about the dangers of dieting, who cared? It wasn't until much later that we realized our food games could kill us.

WISE WORDS

Bulimia is an eating disorder manifested through abnormal eating habits. It primarily affects women, who get into a vicious cycle of gorging huge amounts of food and then making themselves vomit or taking laxatives to get rid of the food.

Bulimia, a psychological disorder exhibited through abnormal eating habits, usually hits people between the ages of 17 and 25, although often they are not diagnosed with it until their 30s. People who see themselves as "failed" anorexics often turn to bulimia for more effective results. A study showed that the incidence of bulimia from 1980 to 1983 tripled from 1 to 3 percent of incoming university freshmen women.

The Causes and Effects of Bulimia

Unlike most anorexics, who usually starve themselves, bulimics eat huge amounts of food. After bingeing, however, they get rid of extra calories by purging what they've eaten through vomiting, abusing laxatives, or exercising obsessively. Why do bulimics engage in bingeing-purging cycles? Many women become bulimic because that's a way of dealing with their anxiety, frustration, loneliness, and other personal problems.

Bulimic binges can last between one or two hours, and many girls consume between 15,000 to 20,000 calories of junk food in one binge! Others may binge on healthy foods. A dietitian told us that one patient binged on a whole chicken or a loaf of bread.

Bulimia doesn't lead to starvation, but it has serious consequences:

- Constant vomiting erodes the esophagus, the gums, and the teeth.

- Vomit-inducing chemicals may also rip the esophagus, a rare but potentially fatal complication.

- Constant vomiting can also lead to dehydration, loss of potassium, and kidney damage.

ALL IN THE FAMILY

 Throwing up is the most common method of purging food. Some bulimics gag themselves by sticking their fingers, spoons, or other objects down their throats. Others swallow *emetics*, chemical substances that cause vomiting. Bulimics think their retching will get rid of calories, but experts say they are wrong: Vomiting mostly gets rid of water.

What to Watch for

Your daughter may be bulimic if she is:

- Discontent with her body and thinking that being thin could change her life

- Having recurrent episodes of binge eating (consuming huge amounts of food)

- Resigning herself to the fact that her eating pattern is abnormal but not being able to change it

- Repeatedly purging, dieting, or vigorously exercising

- Bingeing at least twice a week for at least three months

- Repeatedly losing then gaining about 10 pounds from constant bingeing and purging

You can't tell your daughter is bulimic just by the way she looks. Most bulimics can hide this disorder from their families and the public because their weight is typically normal. One way you can tell something is wrong is if you notice that you're going through more groceries than usual.

BINGE EATING DISORDER

Like bulimics, *compulsive overeaters* also binge, but they don't purge right afterwards. As a result, compulsive eaters are usually overweight or obese. About two percent of adolescents and adults have binge eating disorders. Compulsive overeaters don't have any control around food. Because they can't moderate what they eat, they often binge in secrecy—and feel guilty about it. Compulsive overeaters tend to be depressed and, because of their high fat intake, at higher risk for heart disease.

WISE WORDS

People who are *compulsive overeaters* don't starve themselves (as do anorexics) or get rid of food by purging (like bulimics). Most people with this disorder are overweight.

COPING WITH FOOD DISORDERS

You may rule the roost at work and control what your family does during vacation, but you can't handle your kid's eating disorder on your own. Treating eating disorders requires a team effort: a psychotherapist who will help your child figure out the emotional causes of the disorder, medical doctors who'll monitor your child's physical well-being, and nutrition counselors who'll help devise diets to get your kid back on track.

Whether your child is anorexic, bulimic, or a compulsive eater, she'll have to do the following:

◆ Be medically stabilized or even hospitalized if she has a dangerously low body weight or has been doing so much vomiting that her body chemistry is distorted.

◆ See a mental health professional for some time (because eating disorders are mostly mental disorders).

◆ Work with mental health professionals, who will coordinate treatment along with doctors and dietitians.

Different eating disorders require different ways of changing eating patterns. But remember, these disorders are complex and you can't change your child's eating behavior alone. You must seek the help of a dietitian. Here's a general idea of what to a dietitian may recommend for your child.

◆ Anorexic kids need to change their pattern of undereating so they can gain weight and keep it at a normal level.

◆ Bulimics must eat more during meals and snacks so they don't starve themselves and then binge later.

◆ Compulsive eaters must eat moderately during meals and stick to healthful snacks during scheduled times.

Feeding Your Anorexic Child

Your anorexic child must first recover her weight. Her dietitian will determine how much she should weigh based on pediatric charts as well as caloric requirements. She'll need to eat extra calories to recover. If she exercises during this period, she must make up the calories she burns by eating more. When she reaches her goal weight, her daily caloric requirements can be changed to the level that will maintain the right weight for her.

To see how your daughter is doing, have her weigh herself at the same time every day, preferably with as little clothing on as possible. The best time is first thing in the morning after urinating. After she has pumped herself up with enough calories, her dietitian will probably suggest an eating plan that allows her to spread calories through the day at meals and snack time.

MOM ALWAYS SAID

Be prepared to run up against resistance when your anorexic child is in recovery. Remember, an anorexic child doesn't want to eat. What your child eats is something your child and her dietitian have to decide on. The feedings won't be rigid, so they can be adjusted to fit your child's lifestyle. Don't count exact calories. Instead, emphasize numbers of servings and types of foods.

Your child may also need some vitamin and mineral supplements to help restore nutrients that have been depleted during the starvation phase of anorexia. Talk to your child's doctor or dietitian.

Feeding Your Bulimic Child

The recovering bulimic child may not have to gain or lose weight. Mostly, she needs to know what she should eat (in terms of calories and serving sizes) to maintain her weight. Like anorexics, though, bulimic children are afraid they'll gain weight if they eat normally.

Generally, bulimics and anorexics require the same treatment:

◆ Set weight goals, caloric requirements, and exercise goals.

◆ Establish meal patterns on a case by case basis.

◆ Eat three meals a day; each one should have the same amount of food to prevent the feeling of overeating anytime.

Treating a child with bulimia is not just a matter of making sure she eats the right things. The problem is much more complex and requires your daughter to change her mentality her approach to eating. Again, don't try to help her on your own.

Helping Your Binge Eater

If you don't have any eating disorders yourself, teach your binge-eating child to eat in response to hunger until she feels full. She will have to eat fewer calories and have a more regular eating schedule. Dietitians will work with your child to help promote behavioral changes by suggesting the kid play a game, ride a bicycle, or join a soccer team, for example, to take her mind off food. If you do have an eating disorder, get help before you try to help your child, to avoid inadvertently passing on negative eating messages.

MOM ALWAYS SAID

Don't try to be superwoman when you've got an anorexic or bulimic daughter on your hands. It's not just your child who needs help to cope with the disorder—you do too. You may have thought life was fine before your daughter was diagnosed, but obviously your daughter didn't think so. Recovery is bound to unearth some negative feelings about your family interactions, but you have a chance to show her how much you love her and that you are willing to do what it takes to help her.

PREVENTING EATING DISORDERS

So far, I've talked about what you can do to help a child already afflicted with eating disorders. But what can you do to prevent them? Author Ellen Satter says parents and children must have a "positive feeding relationship, where the mom offers healthful foods and the child chooses to eat or not to eat."

Here are some other prevention pointers:

◆ Develop healthy relationships at home. You and your spouse, says Satter, have to get along well with each other and leave out the children when you are fighting. Many families, she says, have unhealthy relationships and don't realize it. According to Satter, if your children are not doing well, something is going on at home. Developing an eating disorder is only one of the symptoms your child might show.

◆ Model healthier eating yourself. Your daughter will probably mimic your eating style. If you grab food on the run, drink lots of soda, and eat high-fat foods, and then go on a crash diet, this pattern is what will seem normal to your daughter, and what she'll want to do as well. If you can't rely on what Satter calls "internally regulated eating," then seek help, for your daughter's sake.

◆ Don't put your kid on a diet. Don't tell your child, "stop eating that," or "no, you'll gain weight if you put that in your mouth!" Instead, teach her to regulate her food intake based on her internal cues of hunger and appetite.

◆ Tell your child to wait 20 minutes to see whether she is still hungry. If so, then she should eat something then.

◆ Change the standard: Everyone is beautiful. In this society, children are terrified about becoming obese. Unless they are as thin as models and superstars, they won't feel they can be "beautiful." But that standard is unrealistic and totally out of whack with how our bodies look. One humorist, Satter points out, said that if Miss America continues to get thinner, she'll be dead in another 20 years.

YOUR DAUGHTER, YOURSELF

According to Eating Disorders Awareness & Prevention, Inc., parents can follow these tips to help prevent eating disorders:

◆ Look at how your beliefs, attitudes, and behaviors about your own body have shaped your opinions of your child's body. Then educate your kids about the genetic basis of differences in body types and the prejudices society has about anyone who isn't picture-perfect thin.

◆ What are your goals and dreams for your kids? Are you overemphasizing beauty and body shape? Avoid conveying an attitude that says, "I will like you more if you lose weight, don't eat so much...". Do what you can to stop yourself from teasing or blaming overweight children and glorifying slenderness. Also stop making comments about other people's children being overweight. When talking about people, focus on what they are like, rather than how they look.

◆ Teach your kids the dangers of dieting, the value of moderate exercise just to feel your body move, and the importance of eating a variety of foods at meals at least three times a day.

◆ Don't avoid swimming, dancing, or other exercises just because these call attention to your weight and shape.

CALL FOR HELP

If you need information and referrals for treatment of eating disorders, call the organizations listed below. But again, discuss your child's problem with an MD first. This is not a disorder you can treat yourself. If you can't find a dietitian, you can call the American Dietetic Association, which will direct you to professionals in your area.

National Association of Anorexia Nervosa & Associated Disorders
P.O. Box 7
Highland Park, IL 60035
(847)831-3438

American Anorexia/Bulimia Association, Inc.
(212)575-6200

Eating Disorders Awareness and Prevention, Inc.
603 Stewart Street, Suite 803
Seattle, WA 98101
(206)382-3587

National Eating Disorder Organization
Laureate Eating Disorder Unit
6655 South Yale Avenue
Tulsa, OK 74136
(918)481-4044

THE LEAST YOU NEED TO KNOW

- ◆ Eating disorders affect 10 to 15 percent of middle and high school girls.

- ◆ Anorexia nervosa involves self-induced starvation and can be life threatening.

- ◆ Bulimia involves repeatedly gorging on food, and then purging it by vomiting or using laxatives or diuretics.

- ◆ Compulsive overeaters tend to be extremely overweight because they binge but do not purge.

- ◆ Different eating disorders require different treatments, but all treatments call for a team of experts working with your child, including a medical doctor, psychologist, and a dietitian.

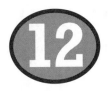

Food Sensitivities

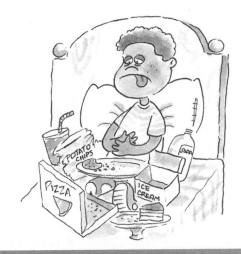

When it comes to food allergies, everyone's an expert. Their child's stomach hurts, they say, "Oh, he's allergic to milk." Their daughter races to the bathroom after eating pasta and bread; they think, "She may have a wheat allergy." They even blame their kids' grumpy moods on pollen allergies and hay fever. But the experts say that most kids don't have allergies. Instead, many kids suffer from *food intolerance* that can be treated by partial or total removal of the foods that make the children miserable. This chapter looks at how allergies differ from intolerance and what you can do to give your child proper nutrition. I'll also explain how you can get your child tested for allergies.

FOOD ALLERGIES: SCRATCH, SNEEZE, AND RACE TO THE JOHN

Allergies exist, but they are much less common than you might think. According to the *Yale Guide to Children's Nutrition* (Yale University, 1997), research shows that of parents who were convinced that their children had a food allergy, only 39 percent actually did.

A *food allergy* occurs when your child's immune system makes a mistake and attacks the good proteins in his body (the ones mending his tissue). Put on the offense for no good reason, his body prepares for war, producing antibodies to kill the innocent proteins. The body releases chemicals, like *histamine*, to irritate the tissue. The results? Your child may feel nauseated, develop skin rashes, have difficulty breathing, have diarrhea, or vomit. In other words, your child will experience the same symptoms he has when he feels sick. (In fact, if your child does get sick, a doctor who can't find anything wrong with him may just blame it on allergies.)

Most of the foods that cause this type of reaction (90 percent) are harmless, wholesome everyday foods he'd eat at grandma's, such as protein in cow's milk, egg whites, peanuts, wheat, shellfish and soybeans. And how long after you eat foods you're allergic to do you feel sick? Usually within two to four hours after the food was consumed. The most severe reactions can take place within minutes.

WISE WORDS

A *food allergy* is an inappropriate reaction of the immune system to a food. Common food allergies include sensitivity to cow's milk protein, wheat, fish, shellfish, and eggs. Allergic reactions—which include vomiting, abdominal distention, diarrhea, and other symptoms—usually take place within two to four hours after the food has been eaten.

If you think your child has a food allergy, you can either dabble in alternative health medicine and try a natural cure—but be sure to do a lot of research first—or get a diagnosis from a physician certified by the American Board of Allergy and Immunology. Ask your primary doctor for a referral to a certified physician or call the

American Academy of Allergy and Immunology at 1-800-822-2765 and they'll refer you to physicians in your area.

These physicians know the nuance of every itch, sneeze, and scratch your child may get from food allergies, and they'll prick and stick your child until they get to the source of the problem.

If your child has difficulty breathing, is wheezing, or breaks out in hives, you should make sure he is examined.

MOM KNOWS BEST

Some research shows that chocolate does not cause allergic reactions. And, all those years we spent as teenagers worrying that chocolate, sugar, and greasy french fries were the cause of our pimples? We were wrong there too. Most dermatologists haven't linked an underlying relationship between acne and diet.

THE PROBE AND PRICK TEST: DIAGNOSING FOOD ALLERGIES

If you arrange an appointment with an allergist, you can expect the allergist to ask about the following:

◆ Your family medical histories

◆ When and how often your child gets the allergy symptoms

◆ What your child eats when the symptoms show up

The allergist will also do a complete physical, specifically examining the condition of your child's skin, eyes, and the inside of her nose and mouth.

You may be asked to keep a diary documenting every bite your child takes and recording when her symptoms start. If you are not with her all day, get her teachers and caretakers to handle the reporting. If your kid is old enough, she may want to do the recording herself.

If the doctor still can't figure out what's making your child sick, he or she may ask your child to follow a *restrictive-elimination diet*, in which all suspicious foods are banned from your child's diet.

Each food will then be re-introduced slowly, one at a time, so you can identify which one is the culprit.

Prick Them with a Needle

If the elimination plan doesn't work, your allergist may recommend that you take your child for a skin test. In a skin test, a doctor drops liquid extract of individual foods on a section of your child's arm or back and then sticks, scratches, or pricks the area. If itching or swelling appears within 20 minutes, she may be allergic to that food. Skin tests are not 100 percent reliable. Some kids develop skin rashes even though they are not allergic to the extracts splattered on them, and other children don't show any physical reaction even though they are allergic. So why would anybody want to try this test? Beats me. But if you have no clue as to what's wrong with your kid, you'll try anything!

Tests, Tests, and More Tests

If everyone is still baffled, the next diagnostic tool is the *RAST Test* (Radioallergosorbent tests). Medical professionals draw your child's blood and mix it with food extracts. If she's got a food allergy, her blood sample will contain additional allergy antibodies. Some say the RAST test is less accurate because the substances are mixed outside your child's body. On the other hand, it's a great test because if your child is indeed allergic to the food, she won't have to live through yet another allergic reaction to find out.

Bet on the Double-Blind Challenge

Another test to identify food allergies is the *double-blind challenge* test. The child is given two types of capsules to take. One contains nonreactive substances; the other has one type of food that she may react to. Nobody knows which capsule has what. If your child develops symptoms after taking the stuffed capsule, you've found the cause of the allergy. If she has a reaction after taking the empty one, well, it's time to tell her that nothing's wrong with her, allergy-wise.

COMMON FOOD ALLERGIES

Milk proteins, eggs, and wheat are the most common causes of food allergies. Because these ingredients are found in most of the foods we eat, if you suspect your child is allergic to any of them, you'll have to start reading food labels very carefully. For your first trip to the store to get egg-free products or wheat-free pastas, do yourself a favor. Leave rowdy children at home and be prepared to read a lot of very long words that you'll never be able to pronounce.

Milk Allergies

It is believed that .5 percent to 3 percent of all children are allergic to cow's milk. Most studies show that at least one-third of all kids outgrow cow's milk allergies by the time they turn three, but unfortunately, others stay allergic to cow's milk for a long time.

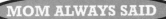

MOM ALWAYS SAID

Don't confuse cow's milk allergies with *lactose intolerance*, which is discussed later. They are two separate conditions.

The level of sensitivity varies from kid to kid. Your child may not be able to drink cow's milk, but he might be fine with small portions of cheese or yogurt. Others can tolerate milk so long as it's heated. Other children may not be able to drink cow's milk or any of its by-products. Because cow's milk is one of the main sources of calcium, protein, riboflavin, and vitamins A and D, make sure your child eats other nutrient-rich foods to make up for the loss. Some older kids can drink goat's milk. Goat's milk doesn't have enough folic acid, however, so your kid may need to get this nutrient from other foods or take supplements. Children with allergies to milk's protein may also be able to drink soy milk, but, as usual, check with your child's nutritionist or dietitian.

If your child cannot stomach any milk or milk products, you'll need to make sure he gets enough calcium from other sources (remember, teens need about 1,200 milligrams of calcium a day). Calcium can come from the following sources:

◆ An eight-ounce glass of calcium-fortified orange juice (300 milligrams of calcium)

◆ An ounce of calcium-fortified cereal, such as Total (250 milligrams)

Of course, you shouldn't serve your allergic child milk products like butter, ice cream, yogurt, or pudding. But other foods that contain milk are not so obvious. Avoid foods that mention the following milk by-products on the ingredients list:

◆ Buttermilk

◆ Casein

◆ Caseinate

◆ Condensed milk

◆ Cream

◆ Curds

◆ Lactose

◆ Powdered milk

◆ Sodium caseinate

◆ Whey

Feeding a child who is allergic to cow's milk isn't easy. You always have to be on the lookout to ensure he is getting his protein (if milk substitutes are not used) and calcium requirements from somewhere else. Your kid still needs many different foods to get all his nutrients, including one or two servings per day of protein-rich sources like eggs, meat, poultry, fish, or legumes.

Egg Allergies

If your child is allergic to eggs, you'll know about it shortly after he takes his first bite. The first signs may be itching and swelling in his mouth—followed by progressive difficulty breathing, along with coughing, wheezing, and chest tightness.

Unfortunately, the cause of egg allergies is the white part of the egg—the part that has no cholesterol or fat and plenty of protein. Luckily, your child can eat plenty of other high-quality protein foods, such as meats, fish, and poultry. Your child can also eat potatoes and rice (so long as there is no egg in it), most commercial and homemade breads, crackers, and other favorites—as long as no eggs are in its ingredients. But he should probably stay away from hot breads like muffins and French toast (unless made without eggs or with substitutes), custard, some soups, and some salad dressings.

The problem is that egg by-products are everywhere; they're hidden in cakes, cookies, breads, and sauces. They are the busy little worker bees that thicken and bind ingredients together so that a piece of cake doesn't disintegrate in your hands. So what's a mom to do?

First, you can use egg-free substitutes—found in supermarkets in the dairy section or freezer—in many recipes. But be aware that these substitutes may have some cholesterol—and don't confuse these with egg beaters which have eggs in them, but no cholesterol.

Another option, as suggested by the writers of *Parents' Guide To Nutrition*, is to replace eggs used to thicken liquid ingredients by combining two tablespoons of whole wheat flour, one half a teaspoon of oil, one half teaspoon of baking powder and two tablespoons of milk, water or fruit juice to replace each egg.

MOM ALWAYS SAID

Before you fill up your cart with egg-free substitutes, read the labels carefully to ensure the brand you buy doesn't have egg whites (called *albumin*).

Your child can also enjoy many products right off the shelf. Many breads, soda crackers, graham crackers, and cereals are made without eggs. If your daughter feels left out because she can't eat certain desserts, tell her she can still have sherbet, frozen yogurt, and other sweet foods.

If your child has an egg allergy, don't worry. It's not the end of the world. Thanks to egg-less products, there is almost nothing you can't make to satisfy your child's nutrition needs and sweet palate. But it's crucial that you check food labels to make sure eggs are not listed in the ingredients.

Wheat Allergies

If your kid races to the bathroom after eating cakes, doughnuts, and pastas, he could be allergic to wheat. "Oh my God! Isn't that like being allergic to air?" you may be thinking. Although it's true that wheat flour is an ingredient in most common products, many companies now make wheat-free alternatives.

Kids who are allergic to a component of wheat called *gluten* have *celiac disease* or *celiac sprue* (formally called *gluten enteropathy*). In this condition, an extract of gluten, called *gliadin*, harms the gastrointestinal tract. As a result, your child can't absorb nutrients. This condition could impact your child's growth and trigger diarrhea.

Some kids get this condition earlier than others, and the symptoms also vary from kid to kid. But most kids with celiac disease start getting diarrhea between 6 and 24 months of age, although many don't get diagnosed until their adolescence or adulthood. After all, the symptoms are not that different from those your child gets from an upset stomach—and it's easy for parents to assume their kids have a stomach ache "from eating all that junk." But, as with all allergies, parents should work with a physician or a registered dietitian when their kids have allergic reactions. To get more information on celiac disease call the Celiac Disease Foundation at 1-818-990-2354.

When gluten is removed from diet, kids with celiac disease are fine and ready to rock and roll, but to stay in good health, they must remain on a gluten-free diet forever.

> **MOM KNOWS BEST**
>
> Because wheat flour also comes loaded with iron, thiamin, niacin, and riboflavin, kids on a wheat-free diet must get these nutrients through other foods and possibly supplements. They will also probably need more B vitamins, iron, and fiber, which are nutrients found in most breads and cereals. To make sure your wheat-free kids are eating a well-balanced diet, contact the American Celiac Society for recipes, wheat-free product information, and meal planning.

Wheat products most likely to trigger allergic reactions include the following:

- Baked beans
- Cakes, candies
- Canned soups with noodles
- Cheese spreads and sauces
- Doughnuts and doughnut mixes
- Pretzels
- Waffles, pancakes
- Muffins
- Chili con carne
- Foods made with enriched flour, hydrolyzed flour, MSG, and sodium glutamate

Also, avoid foods made with the following by-products of wheat:

- Gluten
- Bran
- Food starch
- Hydrolyzed vegetable protein
- Wheat germ
- Vegetable gum

LACTOSE INTOLERANCE: HORSE OF A DIFFERENT COLOR

If your kids complain about having a tummy ache or a gassy stomach after drinking milk or eating a milk product, you may think they have a milk allergy. Although it's true that they are having an adverse reaction to milk, the cause usually is *lactose intolerance*, not an allergy. Allergies affect the body's immune system. *Food intolerance*, on the other hand, usually affect the body's metabolism, which is unable to digest the foods.

Lactose Intolerance: Indigestible Dairy

Kids with lactose intolerance don't make enough of an enzyme called *lactase*, which is needed to digest *lactose*, a *disaccharide*—simple carbohydrate or sugar—found in milk. So when they drink regular milk or dairy products, they get gas, diarrhea, cramps, and bloating.

How do kids get this condition? It's just another one of those dandy things you've passed down to them, along with fat genes, phobias, and dozens of other problems that make family therapists rich. Lactose intolerance is hereditary and strikes people from all over the world. In fact, between 30 to 50 million Americans may suffer from some degree of lactose intolerance.

The condition also affects everyone differently. Your daughter may take a sip of milk and groan all morning about a stomachache. Your son, however, could drink a half a glass of milk and be in fine shape to meet his friend at Starbucks a half an hour later.

ALL IN THE FAMILY

If you aren't sure whether your kid has a milk allergy or *lactose intolerance*—and your doctor isn't either—your doctor may use a hydrogen breath test to check it out. When food containing lactase is *not* digested (as is the case with lactose-intolerant people), hydrogen gas is produced, and its rate of expiration can be measured from the mouth. The more hydrogen gas your child produces, the more lactose-intolerant he may be. But if the doc is tuned in to your son's allergy, he'll probably just remove the culprit food and see if the symptoms go away.

Life in the Lactose Lane

Lactose intolerance doesn't have to turn your family's life upside down—or right side up if it's already chaotic. It all depends on how severe your child's lactose intolerance has become. Here are some tips on feeding lactose-intolerant children:

◆ Your lactose-intolerant child may not keel over with stomach pain if she eats yogurt because the bacteria in yogurt produces lactase, which breaks down the milk sugar on its own.

◆ Watch portions. Downing a glass of milk may do your preteen in for the day, but she may be OK with a little bit of milk added to cereal. An extra-cheese pizza may upset your child's stomach, but a vegetarian pizza with only a dollop of cheese may be just right.

◆ Your child can try Toffuti or other non-dairy ice cream substitute such as sherbet.

◆ Buy one of everything from the lactose-reduced product section in your supermarket. You can't go wrong with Lactaid milk, Lactaid cottage cheese, and Lactaid ice cream. DairyEase is another popular brand.

◆ You can buy tablets or drops at a supermarket or drugstore to put into regular milk that break down the lactose. The milk is ready for one and all a day later.

◆ Special lactase enzyme pills are also available. If your child can swallow these pills, she can take them before eating or drinking a dairy product. Kids can take these pills with school lunch too. This approach may be particularly helpful if your child is going to a party where everyone is eating cake and ice cream.

ALL IN THE FAMILY

 Do food with sugars, artificial colors, and artificial flavors cause hyperactivity? Is obesity a result of food allergies? If you say yes, you're wrong. Experts from the Mt. Sinai School of Medicine are trying to dispel these and other myths about food. The following statements are not true:

Kids who eat food with sugars, artificial colors, and artificial flavors can become hyperactive and develop other behavioral problems. (Studies show that eliminating foods with these ingredients doesn't help kids with hyperactivity or attention-deficit disorder.)

Kids who are obese or compulsive eaters have food allergies.

Some forms of schizophrenia, manic depression, or chronic fatigue result from eating common foods.

Bed-wetting and premenstrual syndrome (PMS) are caused by certain foods, including those that contain amino acids.

THE LEAST YOU NEED TO KNOW

- Food allergies are not as common as you might think.

- Foods most likely to cause allergies include protein in cow's milk, egg whites, peanuts, wheat, and soybeans.

- If you suspect that your child may have a food allergy, consult an allergist for testing.

- A food allergy affects the immune system. A food intolerance affects only the digestive system.

- Lactose intolerance is the inability to digest lactose, a complex natural sugar found in milk. Symptoms of lactose intolerance include gas, diarrhea, cramps, and bloating.

Wise Words Glossary

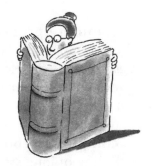

amino acids   A group of 20 chemical compounds that make up all human proteins.

anaphylactic shock   A rare, severe, and life-threatening allergic reaction. The reaction usually happens in response to an insect sting or injected drug.

anorexia nervosa   An eating disorder characterized by fear of being fat, severe weight loss, and eventual absence of monthly periods. Girls and women who suffer from this disorder see themselves as fat even when they are normal weight or emaciated.

atherosclerosis   A disease in which *plaque* forms on the inner lining of the arterial wall, thus narrowing the channel and impairing blood flow. This disease is found most often in people with high concentrations of cholesterol in their bloodstream.

bulimia   An eating disorder characterized by bouts of overeating usually followed by self-induced vomiting. Bulimics usually binge and purge in private, so the illness may not be diagnosed for several years after it has started.

calcium   A mineral that makes up much your bones and teeth, calcium also appears in the soft tissues and body fluids.

calorically dense foods   Foods that pack many calories and fat grams in a small serving size.

calorie   The amount of energy that food provides.

carbohydrates   One of the main sources of energy. Carbohydrates are considered essential in a healthy diet. Sugar and starches are the most familiar types of carbohydrates.

celiac sprue   A condition in which the lining of the small intestine is damaged by gluten, a protein found in wheat, rye, and other cereals. Also known as *gluten enteropathy*.

cholesterol   A fatty substance found in all animal fats, bile, skin, blood, and brain tissues. At elevated levels in the blood, cholesterol is a primary risk factor in cardiovascular disease.

complete proteins   Proteins that contain a good amount of all essential amino acids, found in animal proteins like meat, fish, eggs, milk, or cheese.

complementary proteins   Protein-containing plant foods that are incomplete by themselves but complete when combined. A good example is rice and beans.

complex carbohydrates (complex sugars)   Compounds consisting of long strands of many simple sugars linked together.

daily value   A figure that refers to how much of a day's recommended amount for a certain nutrient is supplied in one serving of a food product.

dehydration   A condition in which the body's water content plummets to a dangerously low level.

eating disorder   One of a range of psychological problems affecting mostly women. The two most common eating disorders are *anorexia nervosa* and *bulimia*.

empty calories   Calories with no nutritional value.

enzyme   Protein molecules that trigger chemical reactions taking place in our bodies.

essential amino acids   Amino acids that are not made in the body and must be taken in from outside food sources.

fat   Nutrients that provide the body with the most concentrated form of energy (one gram of fat has 9 calories). Chemically, fats consist mostly of fatty acids combined with an oily alcohol called glycerol. Fats are divided into *saturated* and *unsaturated*.

fat-soluble nutrients   Nutrients that dissolve in fat. Fat-soluble nutrients include vitamins A, D, E, and K.

food allergy   An overreaction by the body's immune system, usually set off by protein-containing foods like cow's milk, nuts, soybeans, shellfish, eggs, and wheat.

food intolerance   An adverse reaction by the body to foods that don't affect the immune system. Lactose intolerance one such example.

food sensitivity   A catch-all term that includes food intolerances, food allergies, and any other abnormal reactions to food or food additives.

fructose   A naturally occurring fruit sugar.

glucose (dextrose)   The body's chief source of energy for cell metabolism. Glucose is a simple sugar and is found in fruits, honey, and vegetables.

gluten   One of the proteins found in wheat and other grains that gives dough its elastic character. Celiac sprue, a sensitivity to gluten, is believed to affect between .1 and .2 percent of the population.

heart disease   A cardiovascular disease almost always caused by atherosclerosis, a hardening of the arteries in which fatty deposits build up on the inner walls of the arteries, blocking the blood flow to the heart muscle.

homogenized milk   Milk that has undergone processing to reduce the size of milkfat globules so the cream doesn't separate. As a result, the milk stays smooth.

hypertension   The medical term for high blood pressure.

incomplete proteins   Proteins found in vegetables, legumes, nuts, and grains, that lack one or more of the essential amino acids.

iron   The best known trace mineral, whose deficiency is widespread.

lacto-vegetarians   Vegetarians who do not eat meat, poultry, seafood, or eggs. They do eat dairy products, however.

legumes   Foods like dried beans, peas, lentils, and bean curd. Many legumes are good sources of protein, iron, zinc, magnesium, and B vitamins.

monounsaturated fats   An unsaturated fat that may help lower blood cholesterol, typically found in olive, peanut, sesame seed, and canola oils, as well as avocados.

obesity   A condition in which a person is 10 to 20 percent above the ideal weight for his or her height.

osteoporosis   A condition caused by a combination of genetic, hormonal, nutritional, and other factors in which bones lose mass and become fragile, brittle, and more vulnerable to fractures.

ovolacto-vegetarians   Vegetarians who do not eat meat, poultry, or seafood, but who do consume dairy products and eggs.

plaque   Build-up of materials along the inner lining of the arteries that can block the passage of blood to the heart.

polyunsaturated fats   Fats from corn, soybean, safflower, sunflower, and sesame seed oils that can also help lower blood cholesterol.

proteins   Large molecules made up of hundreds or thousands of amino acids linked to form long chains. Our bodies need protein to facilitate chemical reactions, help fight illness and disease, transport oxygen all over the body, regulate many body functions, repair tissue, and perform many other tasks that help our bodies grow.

saturated fats   The devil of all fats; responsible for raising your blood cholesterol, paving the way to heart disease. Saturated fats get solid or hardened at room temperature and are mostly found in animal and milk fats.

semi-vegetarian   Vegetarians who do not eat red meat, but do eat chicken or fish once in a while. They also eat dairy products and eggs.

simple carbohydrates   The most basic carbohydrate, made up of simple sugars like honey, jelly, and soft drinks.

sodium   A trace mineral that helps keep your body fluid in balance. Sodium is found in salt and processed food; too much can be harmful to your health.

starch   Found in grains, vegetables, breads, seeds, legumes, and beans. Starch is found in complex carbohydrates that come from plants.

trans-fatty acids   This type of fat is created when unsaturated fats go through a manufacturing process called hydrogenation.

unsaturated fats   Fats composed of either mono-unsaturated or polyunsaturated fats.

vegans   Vegetarians who don't eat any animal products, including eggs or dairy. Their basic diet is plant food products: grains, legumes, fruits, vegetables, nuts, and seeds.

water-soluble nutrients   These are stored and carried by the water in our system. Water-soluble vitamins include vitamin C and the many B-complex vitamins.

Resources

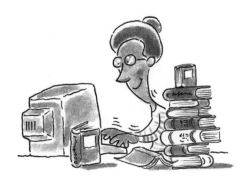

Dr. Attwood's Low-Fat Prescription for Kids, Charles Attwood. Penguin Books USA Inc., 1995.

Eat for Life, the Food and Nutrition Board's Guide to Reducing Your Risk of Chronic Disease, Catherine E. Woteki, Ph.D., R.D. and Paul R. Thomas, Ed.D., R.D. Institute of Medicine, National Academy of Sciences, 1992.

How To Get Your Kid To Eat...But Not Too Much, Ellyn Satter. Bull Publishing Company, 1987.

Parents' Guide to Nutrition: Healthy Eating From Birth Through Adolescence, Susan Baker, M.D., Ph.D. and Roberta R. Henry, R.D. Boston Children's Hospital, 1986.

Play Hard Eat Right, Debbie Sowell Jennings, M.S., R.D., and Suzanne Nelson Steen, D.Sc., R.D. American Dietetic Association, 1995.

The PDR Family Guide to Nutrition and Health. Medical Economics Company At Montvale, N.J., 1995.

The Tufts University Guide to Total Nutrition, Stanley Gershoff, Ph.D. Tufts University Diet & Nutrition Letter, 1990.

The Working Parents' Help Book, Susan Crites Price and Tom Price. Peterson's Career Focus Books, 1996.

The Yale Guide to Children's Nutrition, William V. Tamborlane, M.D., editor. Yale University, 1997.

Total Nutrition: The Only Guide You'll Ever Need, edited by Victor Herbert, M.D., F.A.C.P. and Genell J. Subak-Sharpe, M.S. The Mount Sinai School of Medicine, 1995.

Index

A

adipocytes, 127
amenorrhea and anorexia nervosa, 142
American Academy of Pediatrics (AAP),
    finicky eater categories, 76-78
amino acids, 15-16
anemia and anorexia nervosa, 142
anorexia nervosa
  as step to bulimia, 141
  children, feeding, 147
  defined, 141
  early signs, 143
  percentage of sufferers, 141
  physical effects
    amenorrhea, 142
    anemia, 142
    constipation, 142
    hair loss, 142
    osteoporosis, 142
    percentage of body weight lost, 142
athletes
  caffeinated beverage intake, 108
  caloric intake, 102-103
  carbohydrates as percentage of
    diet, 103
  energy supplements, 106
  fat content in diet, 106
  intake of minerals and vitamins, 106
  meals
    post-event, 112
    pre-event, 110-111
  protein intake, 104
  risk of heat stroke, prevention and
    treatment, 109-110
  sports drink intake, 108
  vegetarians, possible deficiencies in
    diet, 105
  water intake, 107
avoiding
  force-feeding, 73-74
  fried foods, 61

B

B12 vitamin
  danger of deficiencies, 119
  vegetarian intake, 118-119
breads
  as source of starch, 50
  fiber-rich, 50
breakfasts
  alternative recipes, 68-69
  cereals, sugared versus non-sugared,
    68-69
  effect of skipping, 68-69
  importance, 68-69
  ingredients, 68-69
brown-bagging
  desserts, healthy alternatives, 90
  food selections, 88-89
  preparations, 90
  sandwiches, 88-89
  sandwichless lunches, 89
  school lunches, 88-89
bulimia
  bingeing process, 144-145
  caloric bingeing, 144-145
  children, feeding, 148
  defined, 144
  effect of vomiting, 145
  increasing trend, 144
  origins in anorexia nervosa, 141
  physical signs, 145
  typical age range, 144

C

calcium
  food sources, 26
  functions in body, 26
  intake by vegetarians, 119
  RDA requirements, 26